Reflections on Play Therapy

This book explores an extensive range of questions and challenges within the training, theory and practice of play therapy, with the aim of providing a stimulating and thought-provoking debate around many of the issues and dilemmas therapists experience.

Drawing upon the author's own experience as both a therapist and trainer/educator/supervisor, the volume grapples with questions of power, privilege, self-care and mental health. It additionally addresses the wider challenges and impact of the Covid-19 pandemic, climate change and international conflict upon practice and personhood. Questions around training are explored as well as specific practice challenges relating to managing limits and boundaries within play therapy and working with adopted children. Throughout the book, the author will reflect upon aspects of personal and clinical experience, sharing something of his own developmental narrative through training, teaching and practice.

Reflections on Play Therapy will serve as a core text for trainee play therapists and also a valuable resource for any experienced clinicians working therapeutically with children, young people and families.

David Le Vay is a consultant, supervisor and practising independent therapist within a multi-disciplinary therapy team. He worked extensively for many years as a senior lecturer teaching and developing the MA Play Therapy Programme at the University of Roehampton, London.

T0384963

Reflections on Play Therapy

A Narrative through Training, Theory, and Practice

David Le Vay

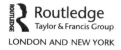
Routledge
Taylor & Francis Group

LONDON AND NEW YORK

Cover image: © Spiderstock via Getty Images

First published 2025
by Routledge
4 Park Square, Milton Park, Abingdon, Oxon OX14 4RN

and by Routledge
605 Third Avenue, New York, NY 10158

Routledge is an imprint of the Taylor & Francis Group, an informa business

British Library Cataloguing-in-Publication Data
A catalogue record for this book is available from the British Library

ISBN: 978-1-032-40332-8 (hbk)
ISBN: 978-1-032-40327-4 (pbk)
ISBN: 978-1-003-35256-3 (ebk)

DOI: 10.4324/9781003352563

Typeset in Times New Roman
by Apex CoVantage, LLC

To Nicky and Jess. This book would not have been possible without you.

Contents

Preface

This book is the culmination of a process that began with *Challenges in the Theory and Practice of Play Therapy*, followed by *Personal Process in Child-Centred Play Therapy*, both edited with my colleague Elise Cuschieri, and like both these books it continues the theme of the personal exploration of some of the challenging questions, debates and dilemmas that lie at the heart of the therapeutic process. But the motivation to write this book also came from the experience of finding myself in a strange period of transition, as I begin to step away from the professional roles that have been so influential in shaping my career. Just as in Chapter 7, where I explore issues around liminality, I find myself now at a threshold between one space and another, and perhaps it is only as I begin to tentatively let go of the reassuring handholds that have for so long anchored me to the security of my professional identity, that I can look back and reflect upon the journey that has led me here.

It is a journey that, like the ever-clarifying focus of a microscope, has brought aspects of practice and experience, the personal and the professional, into sharp, crystalline relief. But *focus* might not quite be the correct word, and although knowing next to nothing about the science of microscopy, I understand there is a difference between *depth of focus* and *depth of field*. The term depth of field seems appropriate in the context of this book. In a technical sense, it refers to the range of sharpness or clarity in front of the lens; in basic terms, the distance between the eye and the object. In a broader sense, we could think of depth of field within a professional context, our particular area of practice, and within this context the process of writing this book has certainly been a deeply personal, immersive experience, as I have sought to explore troubling and challenging questions around the play therapy process; questions of power, privilege, vulnerability and self-care, and what it means to be a 'good enough' therapist. And whilst these are questions that resonate deeply on a personal level, they are questions that I am sure will also resonate widely across the profession; collective, universal themes that are as much about what it means to be human as it does to be a therapist.

Depth of field is also about distance, and I am aware that throughout this book I have taken some risks in exploring these questions from a deeply personal perspective. It is interesting that almost thirty years ago, back in the mid-1990s, when I first trained in play therapy, my research dissertation explored the question of narrative identity; the personal and social stories that we tell about ourselves and others as a way of making sense of our lived experience. True to form, thirty years on, this book is also about narrative identity; a storied account of my journey through my therapist career. Perhaps it is something about transitions, about endings, that also takes us back to the beginning, full circle. Sometimes it is hard to know where one story ends and another begins. And so, albeit rather digressively in places, this book is a narrative account that begins in early childhood and ends in the late, autumn years of my career, reflecting upon key questions, encounters and challenges along the way. It is, I acknowledge, deeply subjective and I have, as they say, rather nailed my colours to the mast in the process, but as a profession we have rightly moved on from the notion of therapist neutrality. The older I have got so seemingly has the line between the personal and the professional become ever finer, and the core attitudinal conditions of my training jostle, sometimes uncomfortably, with the other ethical, moral and political voices that have increasingly sought to make themselves heard.

This is a book primarily about my work as a play therapist, but having also trained in social work, dramatherapy and sandplay therapy, as well as teaching in higher education for over twenty years, I hope that it will be relevant and helpful to people working across these professions and beyond. I also write about some of the very challenging, personal experiences that I have had to negotiate more recently, ill-health and steps towards retirement for example, and again I hope that this will resonate with other people facing similar challenges. On a wider scale, I have also included chapters on my experience of working through the Covid pandemic as well as the very immediate challenge of the climate crisis and the implications this has for child mental health and our work as therapists. Once again, in the context of liminality, it feels as if we are on something of a societal threshold, betwixt and between, and whilst our future remains very uncertain, I think we can say with some certainty that we are living in a period defined by some very considerable existential challenges. My hope for this book as I reflect on some of these challenges is to be stimulating and thought-provoking, provocative perhaps, and to question our role as therapists within a rapidly changing world.

Depth of field then, as we adjust the distance between eye and object, reveals some unexpected parallels and connections, and like the process of heuristic inquiry it is often through the exploration of the personal that we can reveal something of the universal. Like the concentric circles of Bronfenbrenner's model of ecological systems, we flow back and forth, caught up in the societal currents and tides that ebb and flow through our storied lives, taking us to all sorts of unexpected places. Ultimately, narrative inquiry is about curiosity, conversations and shared stories, and I hope that for our field, our therapist profession, this book will add something to the conversation. And whilst writing this book has been a challenging, difficult and at times deeply emotional process, it has also made me appreciate that I have had the rare privilege of learning so much from the children I have worked with, the students I have taught, the deeply influential trainers who taught me, and the supervisors, supervisees and colleagues that have accompanied me throughout my career. This book is a tribute to all of them.

A note on confidentiality

Parts of this book include brief clinical vignettes from the author's practice. Names and identifying details have been disguised, anonymised and pseudonymised in order to protect the identity of those involved. Some of it is composite material. Nevertheless, I am aware that in the course of reading this book you may think you recognise a particular case described. If that is so, I hope that the case depictions are read in the spirit they were written; with the utmost respect for the children and their families and as a way of enhancing our awareness and understanding of the unique process of child-centred play therapy.

Acknowledgements

I would like to thank Grace McDonnell and all at Routledge for their support, guidance and belief in this book.

Thank you also to Lisa Gordon Clark for your time and invaluable feedback.

Finally, thank you to all the children and families who made this book possible and from whom I have learned so much.

Chapter 1

Wherever you go, there you are
Pathways to training and beyond

Introduction

Jack was a tall, rangy, engaging and in many ways very charming young autistic adult. He had a glint in his eye and a mischievous smile, and one could not help but like him. In fact, I came to rather love him. I first met Jack when I started working, in the very early days of my social care career, in a day centre for adults with learning disabilities. This was in the mid-1980s when services for people with learning disabilities still bordered on the edge of institutional, as the larger, longer stay hospitals and institutions (very) slowly began to be closed down in favour of smaller, community-based group homes. I was fortunate to be working in a day centre with a pioneering manager, who challenged the prevailing orthodoxy of the time, was a strong advocate for change and was prepared to take risks. In fact, the key principle and ethos of the service at that time was that of self-advocacy and self-efficacy; supporting and facilitating people with learning disabilities to feel more empowered and to begin to make more choices around the issues that impacted their day to day lives.

I worked in the 'special needs' unit of the day centre, supporting people at the more challenging, acute end of the autistic spectrum, of which Jack was one. His speech was mainly limited to a repetitive echolalia, although within this he had an engaging, rich turn of phrase and endearing sense of humour that was rather infectious. In line with his 6-foot-plus stature, Jack was often very physically active, pacing the corridors of the day centre, whilst at other times, he was prone to deep, extended periods of lethargy and depression, most likely a result of medication. On my first day at work, I was appointed as Jack's new keyworker, a role which I was to continue for the next four years, and it is fair to say that my time spent with Jack was deeply influential in relation to my subsequent training and career in play therapy.

By my new colleagues, Jack was described to me as a 'runner', meaning that he required constant around the clock one-to-one supervision to prevent him from 'escaping' the day centre, placing him at potential risk and vulnerability. Agreeing a rota for 'Jack duty' was a daily part of our work routine, and, of course, being his keyworker much of this responsibility fell to me, happily I would add, and over the

DOI: 10.4324/9781003352563-1

course of the next few years I spent more time in Jack's rather wonderfully quirky, eccentric company than almost anyone else in my life at that time.

It was also around this time that I read the book *Bobby: Breakthrough of an Autistic Child* by Rachel Pinney (1983). Pinney, a medical doctor, can best be described as something of an eccentric of her time, a maverick perhaps and certainly unorthodox in her approaches to child psychology. For a period, Pinney worked alongside Margaret Lowenfeld, the developer of sand-play therapy, and was also strongly allied to, and influenced by, the work of Axline (1989) and the principles of non-directive play therapy, and within this child-centred context Pinney pioneered the approach of Creative Listening and Children's Hours. The principle of the Children's Hour is that within this period, the child is 'free to do whatever he or she may wish, within the bound of danger, damage or impropriety' (1983: 11), whilst the adult gives the child their total attention, is strictly non-directive and is neither encouraging or discouraging, so that the child has the 'experience of having his activity listened to without the intervention of adult views and values' (1983: 12).

Having read *Bobby* and felt inspired by Pinney's radical approach to autism, I proposed to my then manager the rather counter-intuitive suggestion that rather than devoting all our energies to preventing Jack from running away – if that was indeed what he intended to do – we could timetable in a period each day, in keeping with the principle of Pinney's Hour, when he was allowed to go wherever and do whatever he liked . . . in my company. I was curious about his motivation; was it to run or was it to explore? Was it simply about being on the move and a form of self-regulation? One of Jack's stock phrases was 'chase me', because that was the pattern of behaviour that he was familiar with – he ran and people chased – so instead of chasing him, what if I actually joined him on his adventures, as a companion of sorts, explorers together, with my added role of managing limits, minimising risk and facilitating a sense of 'creative containment'?

So, whenever Jack, on whatever impulse, whim or anxious urge was driving him, decided to hit the road, I went with him. In truth, our adventures never took us too far – around the local community and the grounds of the local hospital. We walked together, ran together, sat in fields and played games, sang songs, climbed trees, looked at insects, fed ducks. There was always a degree of managing risk and at times I had to put in limits, which Jack mostly kept to, but there was never a sense of him trying to run away or escape – I guess because he no longer had anything to escape from. This, in the spirit of Pinney, was about an attentive, listening, non-judgemental, permissive state of 'being with' in which we both learned to be in each other's company, to trust each other and know where the limits lay.

I feel deeply indebted to Pinney for her influential role in steering me along the path towards play therapy, and further to this I also feel something of an emotional affinity towards her. She was, like my mother, a quaker and CND activist and I like to think there is a little bit of magical synchronicity between these two formative influences upon my life. In fact, Pinney protested at Greenham Common in the 1980s, as did my mother, and I like to picture them – the communist and the socialist – chained together in body and spirit to the gates of the infamous American airbase. I also feel deeply indebted to Jack. He taught me a lot about autism and the internal landscape of the autistic mind, about the importance of the relationship and emotional connection and attunement, and about the notion of unconditional positive regard, long before I had actually become acquainted with these terms within the context of CCPT. Certainly, like Pinney's adventures with Bobby, I took risks that would be unthinkable now; working on my own with a highly challenging young person, out in the community with no support or mobile phone, but like many behaviourally challenging young children who get referred to play therapy, given an accepting, permissive and emotionally containing relationship, Jack no longer needed to adhere to the familiar patterns of behavioural expectations that were such a defining feature of his daily life.

I share this reminiscence of my time with Jack because, whether or not I knew it then, it was a significant influential factor contributing towards my pathway into play therapy training and practice. For others, it was different; for example, I know that for many it was not Bobby but Axline's seminal book *Dibs: In Search of Self* (1964) that inspired them to train in play therapy. But I would suggest that motivations to train within the field of social care and psychotherapy go back much further than this, to our early, formative childhood experiences, and my aim within this chapter is to explore the question around the kinds of experiences, conscious or otherwise, that might lead people along a path into play therapy and working therapeutically with troubled children. Beyond the oft stated desire to 'care for', 'help', 'understand' or even 'give back' something to children, I am curious about the more unsaid, unknown, psychologically implicit motivations to train. As Barnett puts it, what are the 'unconscious motivations and gratifications for the would-be therapist? What is the shadow side of altruism and how might that affect what happens in the consulting room?' (Barnett, 2007: 257). I will, throughout this discussion, draw upon aspects of my own early childhood experience and also make links to examples from my own current, clinical practice.

Beginnings

I grew up in a rambling old house with a large sprawling, mostly untamed garden on the edge of a small village, set deep within the rich, heady, bucolic countryside of East Sussex. At best, I would describe my childhood as bohemian, certainly unconventional, whilst at worst – and it is interesting to commit this word to writing – rather neglectful. To clarify, I do not mean neglect in any wilful sense, more a process of benign omission. I was a child of the 1960s, a lifetime ago now, and indeed we were very much a family of the time. My father, the child of Jewish immigrants, was an orthopaedic surgeon, writer and translator; a gifted, formidable man, plagued by waves of deep depression and mania. My mother, herself a Danish immigrant, was a nurse and latterly a quaker, political activist, magistrate and tireless charity worker. My father was absent, either in mind or body, for long periods of my childhood. I recall that he could, for brief periods, be an engaging, playful and charismatic father, but was mostly distant and remote, sometimes frightening and often emotionally abusive. It is said that no man is an island; well, my father certainly was.

My mother, struggling (in my father's absence) to feed her ever growing family, worked all the hours she could, in conjunction with her unwavering dedication to social and political activism, invariably involved in all manner of local, national and international campaigns. She was a warm, empathic, deeply caring woman, unstinting in her altruistic commitment to others, albeit perhaps – and again I hesitate to say this – sometimes overlooking the needs of the children at her feet.

I have previously described my childhood as something of a cross between the *Famous Five* (Blyton, 1942) and the *Wasp Factory* (Banks, 1984). Certainly, we were rather feral children, for better or worse. I can recall as a young child spending days on end exploring the local countryside, my parents – unconcerned – having no idea of my whereabouts, their basic parenting principle seemingly an echo of the oft quoted play therapy mantra of 'trust the process'. Both on my own and at times alongside my siblings, I climbed trees, swam in rivers and lakes, built dens in the woods, set things on fire and so on. I also fell out of trees, fell into rivers and lakes, cut, hurt and burned myself. I broke bones – several – was hospitalised on occasion and nearly drowned. And that was just me. Indeed, to this day, a family favourite Christmas game is to try and recall in chronological order all the injuries that we had as children and it is fair to say that it is a formidable list. But all that said, I would not have had it any other way, although, of course, it was all I knew. I was privileged to have the opportunity to immerse myself in the natural world, to explore, take risks, learn about nature, experiment with boundaries, albeit sometimes the hard way. My mother, and by extension our house, provided a secure base from which to explore and return and whilst she was often caught up in having to simply manage from day to day, her love was unconditional.

I have often reflected upon the possible connections between my early childhood, formative experiences and my later decision to train as a therapist and specifically, a play therapist. What motivated me, both consciously and unconsciously, to work therapeutically with troubled children? Was I a troubled child? I grew up in a large family with many siblings; our family home extended in spirit and practice to embrace many others beyond the immediate family. But ironically, being in birth order a 'lower middle' child, I spent much of my childhood playing alone. My constant, unconditional play companions were the wild, rambling acres of garden and the fields, woods, rivers and lakes that extended beyond. In this sense, the natural world of my environment, in which I was totally immersed, became a key attachment relationship. It is interesting to think of attachment beyond the realms of a human, relational phenomenon. Clearly, I had an attachment relationship to my parents, but I was also, I think, attached to a sense of place, with nature taking on the role of a third parent, if I can put it like that, and this ambiguous, amorphous relationship between attachment, place and child development, whilst not explored extensively within literature, has certainly been subject to some interesting research, for example in Little and Derr's (2018) formative study on the influence of nature on children's development and the connections between human and place attachment.

Chawla (1992) defined place attachment as children feeling 'attached to a place when they show happiness at being in it and regret or distress at leaving it, and when they value it not only for the satisfaction of physical needs but for its own intrinsic qualities' (Chawla, 1992: 64). I certainly felt a deep, intrinsic value to my relationship with nature. I knew the garden and surrounding area of my childhood home intimately and, in a sense, it knew me. Every moss-covered flagstone, sculpted branch, fallen tree, hidden nook and cranny, secret place. I knew the stones in the river under which I could catch a Miller's Thumb. I caught newts, frogs, snakes, studied the life cycle of the dragon fly. Within this natural environment, I felt safe, secure and held – even with the risks and dangers that it sometimes presented. Low and Altman (1992) propose that there is an emotional bonding to 'place' – the expression of specific feelings associated with a particular location or place preference, evoking feelings of safety, security and belonging, and a sense of identity and well-being. In short then, an attachment. I particularly recall spending extended periods of my childhood playing by, and in, our large fishpond. It was a wondrous, living, weedy, seething, organic, watery treasure trove of flora and fauna, but more than that it became an extension of my personal emotional world, inexorably linked to my own internal state of being. Indeed, the fishpond, like a relationship, became internalised, like some kind of Kleinian object; a symbolic representation of the 'other'. These special childhood places are held deeply, like the half-lit waters of the pond, within our adult memory. As suggested by Cooper Marcus:

> We hold onto childhood memories of certain places as a kind of psychic anchor, reminding us of where we came from, of what we once were, or of how the environment nurtured us when family dynamics were strained. . . . It is as though childhood is a temporal extension of the self.
>
> (1992: 89)

Research (Lim & Barton, 2010) into environmental memory and the role of children's environments suggests the importance of place not only as a source of outward exploration but also a significant source of inward-focused emotional regulation, places of privacy, self-exploration and gentle introspection. Reflecting upon this now, I do believe that my childhood attachment relationship to my natural environment, be it pond, tree or river, provided places where I could process and explore my thoughts and feelings in relation to what were often very difficult family dynamics. My relationship with 'place' was unconditional, non-judgmental, accepting and permissive – a therapist of sorts – and as Morgan (2010) suggests, the calming, soothing and emotionally restorative qualities attributable to the natural environment are analogous to that of the human care-giver. I recall a feeling of detached emotional reverie, as I played alone within these natural spaces and places, a form of eco-dissociation, one might call it perhaps, and connections can be made with play therapy, for example with the often unconscious and gently dissociative process of a child's sandplay.

Of course, how we understand and define 'place' can vary greatly. Is it about location, geography, memory? Is it something literal or symbolic? Whilst I am talking about place in the context of my childhood experience of the natural environment, for others it will be something – somewhere – very different, and to draw parallels between human and place attachment is potentially problematic, their very different qualities making comparisons difficult. The notion of place suggests a complex and dynamic mix of psychological, emotional, physical, cultural and social factors. As Morgan suggests, the 'sophisticated intersubjective attunement underpinning human attachment has no obvious parallel in place attachment' (Morgan, 2010: 11). No obvious parallel maybe, but then perhaps it is not about the obvious. Whilst not human, it is interesting as to the extent that one might think of place relationship as intersubjective. The environment I immersed myself in was a living, breathing world – a world that provided a secure base from which I could explore, experiment, gain confidence and develop a sense of self. It was a world that required attunement, that calmed me, sometimes threatened me, helped me self-regulate, to feel safe and contained, to process emotion, explore risk and develop resilience, so I would suggest that whilst clearly different from the complex intersubjective qualities of human attachment, my childhood relationship to place was nonetheless a deeply intersubjective experience, embodying many of the qualities that we might consider within the context of attachment theory.

At the heart of this early childhood experience of – and relationship to – a deeply felt environmental sense of place, is also, of course, the role of imaginative play, which brings us back to the connections between early experience and our conscious/unconscious motivations to train as play therapists. As a child, I played with friends and siblings, but as said I often played alone. Going back for a moment to my internalised 'other' of the fishpond, I recall spending hours and days creating dramatic living dioramas – miniature prehistoric scenes with perhaps a great crested newt, with its fiery underbelly and wavy, serrated crest taking the starring role as some great dinosaur or creature from another world. This was small world, projective play; dynamic scenes captured within my held gaze accompanied by complex, unfolding narrative arcs and dramatic storylines. Perhaps, as a child, I was trying to process and make sense of the often-troubling feelings and thoughts I was experiencing. Perhaps I was simply playing. But now, a lifetime later, I sit with troubled children, facilitating their creation of dramatic projective worlds in the sandtray. Maybe I am working as much with myself as I am with the child, our worlds entangled, as my own childhood remembrances intrude – sometimes welcome, sometimes not – into the playroom.

Physician heal thyself

You have suffered sorrow and humiliation. You have lost your wits and have gone astray; and, like an unskilled doctor, fallen ill, you lose heart and cannot discover by which remedies to cure your own disease.

Aeschylus: Prometheus Bound, Trans Smyth, H.W. (1926)

We all, I would suggest, 'lose heart' at times and even perhaps our 'wits' as life invariably seeks to throw us off balance, testing to the limits our capacity to remain resilient and robust. This is part and parcel of the human condition, and perhaps as much as our clients might like to think of their therapists as invulnerable, this is clearly not the case. I know this only too well myself, as I have written about both elsewhere and latterly in this book. Aeschylus' words are suggestive of the notion that as therapists we need to be cognisant of our own emotional wounds; that to be in a position to help others we are also able to help ourselves, to remedy our own ailments, the danger being that otherwise we are vicariously and unconsciously seeking to get our own needs met through the distress of our clients and, as Woskett states, the 'wounded healer may be attempting to immunise themselves against further injury' (1999: 205).

Sussman (2007) considered pursuing a career in psychotherapy a 'curious calling' and Freud, going further, talked of it as the 'impossible profession' (1937). I recall working for many years for a service that provided an assessment and therapy service for children and young people with sexually harmful behaviour; highly traumatised children sexually abusing other children. During one particularly emotionally harrowing case presentation with our external consultant, he reminded us that probably around 98% of the general population had absolutely no experience or knowledge of the kinds of behaviours that we were having to immerse ourselves in on a daily basis. A curious calling indeed. Why was I choosing to do this? What kind of unconscious motivation or psychological impetus was driving me to work in such a challenging area? Was it about unmet need within my own childhood, the experience of 'sorrow and humiliation' as Aeschylus puts it, or was it about something else – status or kudos perhaps – linked to feelings of self-worth, approval and the need to be 'good enough'? Or maybe something else entirely.

These are questions endemic to the 'helping' professions. My experience as a trainer and teacher for many years on an MA Play Therapy training programme has shown me that behind people's initial, stated motivations to want to train in play therapy, there are invariably more complicated stories about trauma, loss and unmet need, and as I have said, I include myself in this. This is why it is so important that personal therapy is a mandatory requirement of the training; so that trainees have the opportunity to explore and reflect upon their own personal process and have the space to address the feelings, thoughts and behaviours that might be evoked through an emotionally tough and intense process of training. But equally, acknowledging and even allowing one's own vulnerabilities into the work can be a real strength, bringing a sense of genuine authenticity to the relationship. These vulnerabilities, often forged in the formative fires of early childhood, are all part of what motivates and brings us to this work, the critical issue being that these motivations are known, explored and brought to conscious awareness, even if not resolved, rather than being dissociatively split off or separated in a way that might detrimentally impact the therapeutic relationship.

References to the 'wounded healer' in literature are numerous, the origins of the term being attributed to Carl Jung (1951). Drawing upon the Greek myth of Chiron, the eldest and wisest of centaurs who bore an unbearable and incurable wound, Jung proposed that 'disease of the soul' was the best form of training for the healer and indeed that it was something of a pre-requisite – that only a wounded physician could heal effectively. In this sense, rather than trying to disown our own troubled histories of loss, trauma and unmet need, to feel shamed by our past, it is the therapist's very experience of being wounded that provides and promotes the potential for deep, profound connection to the client's experience, enhancing opportunities for empathy and attunement and indeed, compassion. The challenge here is about balancing one's own needs with that of the clients, to be able to acknowledge our own personal story, whatever that may be, without overwhelming the process of therapy or indeed the client's own story. The personal process of the therapist (Le Vay & Cuschieri, 2022) is not something to be denied or avoided, but needs to be considered as a significant and indeed inevitable part of the therapeutic encounter, acknowledging the fact that we bring ourselves, our stories and our personhood with us into the playroom. As Yalom writes:

> Patienthood is ubiquitous; the assumption of the label is largely arbitrary and often dependent more on cultural, educational and economic factors than on the severity of pathology. Since therapists, no less than patients, must confront these givens of existence, the professional posture of disinterested objectivity, so necessary to scientific method, is inappropriate. We psychotherapists simply cannot cluck with sympathy and exhort patients to struggle resolutely with their problems. We cannot say to them you and your problems. Instead, we must speak of us and our problems, because our life, our existence, will always be riveted to death, love to loss, freedom to fear, and growth to separation. We are, all of us, in this together.
>
> (1989: 14)

Certainly, as Yalom suggests, we are all in this together and for play therapists, working with the visceral immediacy and directness of childhood trauma, the process is especially challenging given the heady tinderbox of children's transference and powerful projective material. Working with children will inevitably connect with our own developmental experiences of childhood, our experiences of loss, relational trauma, unmet needs around attachment and intimacy, or whatever might be the personal story that has provided the impetus for our pathway into this work. But it may be that for many therapists, and certainly trainees, there might be an avoidance or denial about how early childhood experiences might be a significant factor in career motivation; that it is easier to think about how we might not be 'in this together'. Conversely, people might be cautious about being too open about their past experiences, to avoid criticism, shame or stigma, or accusations of blurred boundaries and of being too close to the work.

But whilst Jung might advocate 'disease of the soul' as a necessary prerequisite for becoming an effective therapist, it may well be that early childhood adversity is not always a positive experience in relation to one's pathway into the profession, and that conversely it might exert a more problematic, negative influence upon professional functioning (Rønnestad & Skovholt, 2003). The question here might be around the extent to which early adverse experiences have been resolved or otherwise, although that is not to say that experiences of early trauma necessarily need to be resolved to be able to train and work as a child psychotherapist. The notion of something being resolved suggests some kind of emotional closure, and if there is one thing we know as therapists it is that early, adverse childhood experiences will always be with us in one form or another. It is a little like unfolding a crumpled piece of paper; the creases and marks, the emotional folds if you like, are always going to remain and forever be a part of who we are, the key being the extent to which one is able to process and reflect upon the feelings and patterns of behaviour associated with these experiences, which are often revisited at key developmental periods in our lives.

And of course, it is not necessarily about early trauma, however that might be defined. As I have said, I spent much of my childhood playing alone, immersed in the vivid worlds of my fervent imagination. Perhaps being one of many siblings I was always somewhat lost, struggling to find my place or a sense of belonging and consequently my character – my personality – has always been marked by a degree of introversion. Interestingly, Barnett's (2007) narrative research study into unconscious motivations to train in psychotherapy found that loneliness, without exception, was a factor for all those involved in the study, and that feelings of isolation were common. Barnett linked this to the issue of intimacy, in the sense of a perceived absence of emotional closeness in childhood; the absence of anyone who was present and available to listen to them, or someone in whom they could confide. So, from an analytical perspective, Barnett suggests that object loss in early childhood creates a sense of narcissistic injury and the subsequent 'need to be needed' (2007: 259), leading to a self-sacrificing motivation to help or heal others. In this sense, Barnett makes a clear link between the motivation to become a therapist and the gratification of unmet need in early childhood.

It is interesting to reflect upon this now. Certainly, I spent a lot of time playing alone, but I am unsure as to the extent to which this connects to feelings of loneliness or isolation. But in terms of attachment, I had a distant father and a pre-occupied mother and, in this sense, I can connect with Barnett's suppositions around intimacy and emotional closeness. Linked to this, it could be said that play therapy, and psychotherapy more generally, is a somewhat solitary profession, certainly intimate within the context of the one-to-one, individual nature of the work and, as Burch (2004) suggested, perhaps many therapists enter into the profession because of a felt sense or need, albeit unconscious, to have contact with people; in other words, that it meets an early unmet need for emotional closeness, connection and intimacy. Interestingly, in the context of my own childhood experience, Barnett's study also highlighted the loss or absence of fathers as a significant factor in the childhood of psychotherapists and counsellors, often compounded by the subsequent emotional absence of the mother through maternal depression. Barnett's study is small, and I would be very cautious about generalising across a wider population, and it would be interesting to look further at the question of childhood paternal absence, particularly for male therapists.

And so, I am curious about my pathway into play therapy, and the extent to which this was informed by early experience. I like to think that my career trajectory was rather a random, haphazard, unplanned meandering of sorts, a story of chance and happenstance. But I wonder if this was truly the case, or whether there might have been more of an unconscious impetus at play. My training and career have taken me from social work, to dramatherapy, to play therapy and finally sandplay. It is a little like focussing the lens on a microscope, a zooming in, going from the macro to the micro, like Bronfenbrenner (1979) in reverse. It is a pathway that has led me, slowly but surely, right back to the inner world of the child, in a sense right back to my 8-year-old self, constructing miniature worlds by the edge of the fishpond. It is as if life's great piece of elastic, stretched to the limit of exploration, has pulled me inevitably back to the beginning. In a sense, as play therapists we are all time-travellers, journeying with children as they return to key developmental stages in their lives; this is the timeless magic of symbolism and metaphor. And of course, this invariably means that we will, on our journeys with children, also revisit key points in our own lives; those 'blue remembered hills' as the poet Alfred Housman (1896) put it. I am also reminded of the image, often seen in science fiction films, of an astrophysicist (usually Jeff Goldblum) demonstrating the space-time continuum and the existence of wormholes by drawing two separate, distant points on a piece of paper and then folding the paper so that the two points are touching, suddenly enabling travel from one connected point to another. Is this not what happens to us sometimes as play therapists within the unconscious process, the countertransfer-ence, as we find ourselves unexpectedly transported back to our childhood selves by these magical acts of remembrance?

Adam and the tower

I recently met with an 8-year-old boy, I'll call him Adam, whose father had left the family very suddenly, leaving him feeling bewildered, hurt and angry. In the first session, he initially wants to throw sand at me and attack me with monsters, the paternal transference communicating his deep-felt anger and distress; would I also reject him, leave him, as his own father had done (and as my own father had done to me?). He then chooses to play Jenga and we start the game in the traditional way, taking it in turns to remove pieces from the bottom of the tower and adding them to the top. But as the structure becomes more unstable, Adam starts to take pieces from the top, fitting them carefully back into the empty spaces at the base of the tower, to stabilise it and make it stronger and more secure.

It is as if he is playing a form of reverse Jenga, and I find myself wondering about his world that so devastatingly collapsed without warning. The empty spaces in the base of the structure feel almost unbearable, symbolic of the painful absence of his father; suddenly, there are great pieces missing from his world and he has to work hard to prevent it from falling apart. As I watch Adam play, endeavouring to secure the tower, I wonder aloud that it feels a little like being an engineer, and Adam tells me his father used to be an engineer and taught him all about it. He goes on to talk about his father's current job, stressing its importance and the fact that his father is 'in charge'. And there it is, the symbolism, the transference, coming into conscious awareness as Adam's intense feelings of loss about his absent father becomes something that can be named and spoken about. But I am also aware of something else: my own 8-year-old childhood self a sudden, unexpected visitor to the playroom – my own childhood wounds burning hot with shame. When I was Adam's age, I could not make sense of my father's absence, his fearful mood-swings and intense unpredictability. What had I done? Was it my fault? Did he hate me? My father's parenting style was often one of humiliation; he sought to demean, a strategy I understand now as a way of relieving himself of his own intol-erable feelings of shame, passed down the line. But even as the emergence of my own childhood memories are unexpected, I think they help me to connect to Adam and his fragile world and to hold onto a sense of paternal empathy. Indeed, we are joined for a moment, connected through our shared loss.

We continue with Jenga and there is a playful tension around which one of us might eventually cause the tower to collapse, our fragile worlds entwined. Adam wants to pour sand over the tower as if testing its capacity to withstand the storm, like some kind of 1970s disaster movie. He experiments with various approaches, angles and pouring devices, the sand lodging in the gaps, crevices and spaces between the pieces, now a shoring up of sorts like mortar in brickwork. He then goes into a lengthy explanation about a magnetic version of Jenga that he has at home, in which both his hands and the pieces are magnetic so that you can control and move the pieces without touching them, linked to an electrode in your brain which enables you to know exactly which pieces to move. He tells me that he can even change the shape of the pieces, turning them into knives so that you can attack people. Who would you attack, I wonder? Superheroes he replies. It is a complex, fantasy narrative about omnipotence and control, and I feel deeply for this child whose world has so completely and so unexpectedly been turned upside down.

The following week, I meet Adam and his mother in the waiting area and he refuses to come to the session. His mother tries to persuade him, and I suggest we just meet for ten minutes or so to see how he gets on but he becomes angry, tearful and increasingly dysregulated, so we agree to leave the session for this week. But I am taken aback by the strength and intensity of his protest. I like Adam, feel an affinity towards him and given the previous session I am surprised at his refusal. There is a part of me that feels hurt, rejected – am I not good enough? I want Adam to like me and feel rather caught up in my own rather self-absorbed process of narcissistic injury. Is this about the good enough therapist? Father? Son? Or indeed mother? Later, I felt unsettled and was struck by my residual feelings of loss, hurt and rejection, as if one of Adam's magically fashioned Jenga knives had become firmly lodged in my gut, puncturing my idealised therapist-self.

The notion of narcissistic injury is interesting in relation to the therapist as wounded healer. Barnett (2007), in her research into the unconscious motivations of those choosing to work as psychotherapists, evokes the classic Greek myth: the story of Narcissus, whose reflected image was one of perfection. The disowned part of the image, the shadow one might suggest, remains both out of sight and out of conscious awareness. As Barnett suggests, 'if the person of the therapist is the instrument of change, it follows that therapists' level of consciousness of their own shadow is of considerable significance' (2007: 260). The notion of narcissistic injury could be thought about as being the result of childhood loss, the child whose sense of self was not validated or appropriately responded to by their early caregivers; the reflected image in the parental pool distorted by the ripples of unmet need. Wilde's story of Dorian Gray (2012) also comes to mind, the idealised image of perfection set against the distorted shadow of the painting, analogous perhaps to Winnicott's (1990) notion of the 'false self'. Again, the emphasis is upon the trainee therapist's need to bring the shadow into view, something of a paradoxical challenge given that by definition, the unconscious lies largely outside conscious awareness. As Barnett says, the potential danger for would-be therapists might lie in 'striving for perfection and a desire to foster an idealized image of themselves to defend against their own limitations and vulnerabilities. Feelings of inferiority and experiences of humiliation may give rise to a need to feel loved and admired' (2007: 261). Adam certainly idealised his absent father, the flawed superhero, and perhaps in the need to maintain the image of him as 'good enough', Adam's feelings of anger, destructive envy and even hate were split off, disowned and redirected towards myself, triggering my own paternal wounds.

Gathering the threads

Beyond the realms of my own personal, anecdotal experience, it would seem that within the research literature (Orlinsky & Ronnestad, 2005; Davies, 2018 etc.) there are some clearly demonstrated links between early relational trauma, unmet need, object (relational) loss and the motivation to train and pursue a career in psychotherapy and, by extension, play therapy. Whilst this may be something that many of us are intuitively aware of, research also suggests that many therapists, particularly trainees, either lack the conscious awareness of these links or deny/ avoid the significance of early childhood experience as a relevant factor towards their career motivation.

A qualitative study undertaken by Davies (2018), exploring this question of motivation, identified six key categories at play: a wounded sense of self; defence of the fragile self; gratification of unmet need; a move from 'other-ish to self-ish'; integration of the self; and liberation of the self. Davies suggests that the first three categories present a 'vicious circle' formed by the unconscious compulsion to repeat or re-enact relational wounds and consequently, she highlights an ethical imperative for therapy trainings to promote an active process of self-reflection, stating that 'those trainings that fail to promote self-reflection in practitioners, or those who resist reflective engagement, are more likely to compulsively loop round the vicious circle, re-enacting a fixer role, which increases the risk of burnout and defensive, unethical practice' (2018: 118). This is important and highlights the very clear responsibility that training programmes have to promote and facilitate reflective, reflexive, experiential learning – including mandatory personal therapy – and that failure to do so would be both professionally unethical and have potentially detrimental outcomes for both therapist and client. Speaking from my own experience of teaching on an MA play therapy programme, whilst trainees may often be initially resistant, avoidant or unaware of the need to fully engage in a process of open self-reflection and exploration, they soon become aware of how critical this process is in the development of their therapist self. As Davies suggests, 'if we have the courage to own, confront, and process triggers and dynamics linked to our disowned relational past and self, rather than concealing them, this will mitigate future defensive practice and facilitate becoming a "Healing Healer"' (2018: 122).

And so, the pathway into training and beyond is a long journey of self-reflection and personal exploration, demanding an ongoing need for self-awareness and self-evaluation. This involves embracing the principle of 'wherever you go, there you are' and an acceptance that we are not able to leave ourselves, our self, behind on this journey and nor should we. Our past is part and parcel of who we are. Like a long-distance hike, we need to be aware of the route; the markers, signposts, cairns, and to not be afraid to look at a relief map, to get a sense of where we are in relation to where we came from, the context, contours, twists and turns of our journey. Working with troubled children will inevitably involve us revisiting troubled periods in our own lives and like Adam and his tower, our very foundations will at times be tested, shaken, pulled out of shape, distorted. Perhaps at times we all have to play Adam's game of reverse Jenga, being aware of where the missing bricks are, the patterns and shapes of absence, and what it is we need to do to try and shore up the shaky structure.

But also, I would suggest that our journey into this work does not necessarily always need to be about trauma, relational wounds and unmet need. It is important to hold on to the notion of play and the creative imagination; that there is a joy to be found in reconnecting with our own playful childhood selves. When I look back on my childhood, I can recognise that yes, there clearly were some very troubled periods and that like my internalised Kleinian fishpond, I escaped into a world of play, imagination and the natural world of my environment as a way of managing these periods, a form of coping strategy, I guess. But I also reflect back upon my playful early years with great fondness and recognise the fantastic resources I had at my disposal. I can draw upon the waters of the pond to sustain and nurture me; the trees, rivers, fields of my childhood are revisited more with a sense of poignant nostalgia than sadness. As the aforementioned, seminal author Iain Banks (2000) once wrote, the soup of life is salty enough without adding tears to it.

Returning for a moment to my walking metaphor, I once hiked the iconic Tour du Mont Blanc, a challenging 170k circular route around the majestic peak of Mont Blanc. What I liked so much about this walk was its very circularity; that it took you back to the beginning, albeit feeling changed, altered, by the experience. Our work as play therapists will invariably take us back to the beginning, both for ourselves and for the children we work with, hopefully leaving both changed by the experience. Time might be linear, but it is also relative, depending upon our frame of reference, and some might even argue that it is circular, and so my aim within this chapter has been to acknowledge the role of our past in shaping both our present and future, and that as therapists our frame of reference needs to encompass our early, formative childhood experiences and how these experiences have influenced our pathways into training and beyond.

References

Aeschylus. Trans. Smyth, H. W. (1926). *Prometheus bound*. Loeb Classical Library Vol 145 & 146. Cambridge, MA: Harvard University Press.

Axline, V. M. (1964). *Dibs; in search of self*. New York, NY: Ballantine.

Axline, V. M. (1989). *Play therapy*. London: Churchill Livingstone.

Banks, I. (1984). *The wasp factory*. London: Macmillan.

Banks, I. (2000). *Look to windward*. London: Orbit Books.

Barnett, M. (2007). What brings you here? An exploration of the unconscious motivations of those who choose to train and work as psychotherapists and counsellors. *Psychodynamic Practice*, *13*(3), 257–274. London: Routledge.

Blyton, E. (1942). *Five on a Treasure Island*. London: Hodder and Stoughton.

Bronfenbrenner, U. (1979). A future perspective. In *The ecology of human development: Experiments in nature and design* (pp. 3–13). Cambridge, MA: Harvard University Press.

Burch, N. (2004). Closeness and intimacy. *British Journal of Psychotherapy*, *20*, 361–371.

Chawla, L. (1992). Childhood place attachments. In I. Altman & S. Low (Eds.), *Place attachment* (pp. 63–86). New York: Springer.

Cooper Marcus, C. (1992). Environmental memories. In I. Altman & S. Low (Eds.), *Place attachment* (pp. 87–112). New York: Springer.

Davies, J. M. M. (2018). *The role of developmental/relational trauma in therapists' motivation to pursue a psychotherapeutic career: A grounded theory exploration*. (Thesis). University of the West of England, Bristol.

Freud, S. (1937). Analysis terminable and interminable. *Standard Edition*, *23*, 209–253.

Housman, A. E. (1896). *A shropshire lad*. London: Kegan Paul, Trench, Trübner & Co.

Jung, C. (1951). *Fundamental questions of psychotherapy*. Princeton, NJ: Princeton University Press.

Le Vay, D., & Cuschieri, E. (2022). *Personal process in child centred play therapy*. London: Routledge.

Lim, M., & Barton, A. (2010). Exploring insideness in urban children's sense of place. *Environmental Psychology*, *30*(3), 328–337.

Little, S., & Derr, V. (2018). The influence of nature on a child's development: Connecting the outcomes of human attachment and place attachment. In A. Cutter-Mackenzie, K. Malone, & E. Barratt Hacking (Eds.), *Research handbook on childhoodnature*. Springer, Cham: Springer International Handbooks of Education. https://doi.org/10.1007/978-3-319-51949-4_10-1.

Low, S. M., & Altman, I. (1992). Place attachment. In I. Altman & S. Low (Eds.), *Place attachment* (pp. 1–12). New York: Springer.

Morgan, P. (2010). Towards a theory of place attachment. *Journal of Environmental Psychology*, *30*(1), 11–22.

Orlinsky, D. E., & Ronnestad, M. H. (2005). *How psychotherapists develop: A study of therapeutic work and professional growth*. Washington, DC: American Psychological Association.

Pinney, R. (1983). *Bobby: Breakthrough of an autistic child*. London: Harper Collins Press.

Rønnestad, M., & Skovholt, T. (2003). The journey of the counselor and therapist: Research findings and perspectives on professional development. *Journal of Career Development, 30*(1), Fall.

Sussman, M. B. (2007). *A curious calling: Unconscious motivations for practicing psychotherapy* (2nd Edition). Plymouth: Rowman & Littlefield Publishers Inc.

Wilde, O. (2012). *The picture of Dorian Gray* (1st Edition). London: Penguin Classics.

Winnicott, D. W. (1990). Ego distortion in terms of true and false self. In *The maturational processes and the facilitating environment*. London: Karnac Books.

Woskett, V. (1999). *The therapeutic use of self: Counselling practice, research and supervision*. London: Routledge.

Yalom, I. D. (1989). *Love's executioner and other tales of psychotherapy*. New York: Basic Books.

Postcards from the playroom

I remember very clearly the first child I ever worked with, post qualifying as a play therapist, back in the mid-'90s. I think every play therapist probably remembers their first child. He was a slight, rather quirky, serious boy with a keen curiosity about the world around him. I wonder now whether he would have been given an autism diagnosis. He apparently had a phobia of vacuum cleaners (zuigerphobia) and when I looked at his referral notes I saw that he was born by ventouse delivery i.e. his birth was assisted by a vacuum cup attached by suction to the baby's head.

I had no idea whether his fear of vacuum cleaners was associated with his vacuum assisted delivery, but there was a hint of this in the referral. Part of me liked to think there could be a connection; it kind of made sense within the context of early, pre-verbal birth trauma, an embodied, somatic memory of being sucked from the womb. Being newly qualified, my mind was filled with Freud, Winnicott and Klein, and you could guess what they would have said (although Freud might have added an element of infantile phallic anxiety). It was easy in those early days to become rather beguiled by interpretation. But more likely his fear of vacuum cleaners was a sensory issue, particularly for a child potentially on the autistic spectrum. Think of it; a strange mechanical machine, deafeningly noisy, being dragged around the house by a stressed parent. Some of them even have faces (the vacuum cleaners I mean), attached to a large elephantine trunk – terrifying. Even our dog would make a mad dash for the door at the first hint of the great, dust-munching beast. And if the dog is scared, hell, I know I need to be scared as well. It would be strange not to fear such a thing.

Albeit twenty-six years ago, I still think of this child now and again as I drag Henry the Hoover around the house like some kind of strange, childhood transitional object. Members of my family would gladly tell you the story that as a young child, my own transitional object of choice was an old, '60s style television ariel, with its two insect-like antennae, that I used to pull along behind me like some kind of weird, pet alien. Little wonder I became a child therapist.

In his sessions the boy loved to dress up as a wizard – he was magical, creative, endlessly inventive. He was a joy to work with and taught me a lot about the power of play. More often than not I have found that the child in the playroom is not the child in the referral. And whilst I am happy to have my mind filled with Freud, Winnicott and Klein et al, I am careful to keep enough space for others.

Chapter 2

Playful pedagogy
The role of reflective, experiential
learning within play therapy training

Introduction

As the prominent philosopher and educational reformer John Dewey stated, 'education is not preparation for life, education is life itself' (Dewey, 1916: 239). Reflecting upon Dewey's words, I often wonder about my own journey through education and the extent to which it either prepared me for life or rather, as Dewey suggests, has been more a part of my experience of life itself. Formally, my early educational years were a rather chequered experience. I scraped through secondary school, failed most of my exams, dropped out early and did not go to university – not that I especially wanted to at the time. I failed school, or perhaps school failed me. Whichever way around, I was certainly taught a lesson in failure that took me some time to recover from. But of course, there is a difference between education and learning; education being a more systemic, formal process aimed towards the development of specific skills and abilities, whilst learning could be thought of as a more informal, continuous, life-long process; more intrinsically motivated and both intentional or unintentional, conscious or unconscious.

Returning to Dewey's words, I do not feel that my early education prepared me much for anything, although I probably learned a lot about myself, and having dropped out of school to join a band (not quite a circus) I then spent my early working years in the residential care sector, supporting adults with learning disabilities, and adolescents in the care system. I was not much older than many of the teenagers I was working with and as I have spoken about in the first chapter of this book, these early formative experiences were most likely (on reflection) the beginnings of my unconscious pathway into becoming a therapist. In an informal way, this period of my life was clearly a learning experience; I may not have got the certificates, but I learned a great deal about who I was, what I wanted and perhaps also what I needed. Having grown up in a large, bohemian, unconventional family, often feeling somewhat lost and unsure quite where I fitted in, it is interesting that I identified so closely with young people in residential care. Later, in my mid-20s, I then revisited the arena of formal education, feeling better equipped, and over a period of years trained in social work, dramatherapy and play therapy.

DOI: 10.4324/9781003352563-2

Reflecting now upon my experience of higher education, I can understand that there was a process at play; a sense of trying to emotionally work something out, or indeed, through. As I have described before, it was a little like focussing a microscope, moving from the macro to the micro; slowly but surely zooming into the detail of what I needed to explore. My social work training addressed issues of safeguarding, social policy, ethics, the meaning of the child within society, the politics of the family, one could say, and if we can take politics to mean the study of power relationships and the meaning this has for both the individual and the group, then I can understand the personal, familial context and meaning that this training held for me. It was the big picture, the edges of the jigsaw puzzle slowly being completed from the outside in. In terms of experiential learning, social work training also requires being on placement, a prime example of learning by doing, and over the course of my training I spent time in frontline child protection teams, community work projects, family centres and residential communities. I was learning about different services, teams and organisations, but also perhaps I was learning about groups, my role within these groups and where I felt I belonged.

Further adjusting the lens of the microscope, my dramatherapy training focussed with more clarity and intensity upon the therapeutic process and meaning of groups; the psychodrama of family relationships and psychodynamics of early life. It was a focus that brought my own experience of relationships into sharp, crystalline relief – the self in relation. Being a full-time trainee it was an intensely immersive experience – a living and breathing of experiential learning, personal therapy and process groups, and whilst it was a deeply challenging training experience it was also deeply rewarding. The jigsaw puzzle was broken up, hidden away, begun again, put back in the box, taken out of the box and sometimes discarded altogether. For a long time there were no clearly defined edges; I did not know if I was working from the outside in or the inside out, or both at the same time, and there was certainly no guiding image on the box to work from. At best there were floating clusters of connections; puzzling clouds revealing barely discernible patterns, images and oblique associations. At worst it was a chaotic fragmentation.

My play therapy training focussed yet further inwards, taking me from the societal, to the group, to the individual and eventually to the child, where I could begin fitting the puzzle pieces back together again, but this time from the beginning and in a way that finally made some kind of developmental sense. In this sense, my experience of higher education was something of a life led backwards, a little like Scott Fitzgerald's (1922) story, The Curious Case of Benjamin Button. But another metaphor comes to mind, that of the popular UK television programme The Repair Shop. Although a rather overly nostalgia-laden formula, what I have learned from this programme is that for any object to be properly restored, it needs first to be lovingly, painstakingly, taken apart; the worn and broken parts repaired or even remade, and then carefully cleaned and gently reassembled. No hurried duct tape, superglue or hopeful bits of string. As the experienced specialists on this programme tell you time and time again, the reason for taking something apart is to understand how it works, and until you understand how it works, you will never know how to repair it and ultimately, put it back together again.

Experiential learning and education for me then, was much more than a preparation for life; it was more a process of revisiting, reliving and re-experiencing. For Dewey (1938), education and learning were viewed as an active, social and holistic process, wherein thought is embedded in action and within the context of the environment, a rejection of the more dualistic approach that saw education as a separation between mind and body. This is the essence of embodied, experiential learning and as suggested by Kuk and Holst, 'experience is the totality of the transaction between thought and action, which can be equated with the knowledge of a person . . . although not all experience is learning, learning itself is inevitably an experience and a reflection' (2018: 154).

So, whilst I may not have travelled the more conventional, academic path into my career, I would argue that my early 'wilderness years' were an invaluable process of experiential learning and reflection, informing my later work as a social worker and therapist. And the irony does not escape me, that I subsequently spent close to twenty years as an educator within higher education. This chapter then, is an exploration of my experience as a teacher, trainer and supervisor, as well as my own experience of being a taught trainee. Specifically, I will explore the question of experiential learning within play therapy training. Whilst child-centred play therapy is often talked about as a process of *being* rather than *doing*, I will argue here that in the context of training, the process of *doing* is invaluable, in the sense of active, rather than passive learning. This includes an integrated process of dynamic, embodied learning with a key emphasis upon personal development and reflexivity. Links will be made to emergent research around movement, neuroscience, creative ideation and the notion of playful pedagogy – the importance of play within learning.

Some thoughts on terminology

I am aware that there are several terms within this chapter that I use somewhat interchangeably; that is, they are conceptually related, often overlapping, but can also be understood as having their own discreet meaning. For the purposes of clarity, it might be helpful to look at the specific definition of terms to get a clearer sense of their use and meaning within this chapter.

Experiential learning

In its simplest sense, experiential learning can be defined as learning through doing. The Association for Experiential Education defines experiential learning as a 'philosophy and methodology in which educators purposefully engage with students in direct experience and focused reflection in order to increase knowledge, develop skills, and clarify values' (AEE: 2). Kolb (1984), with a slightly different emphasis, defined experiential learning as a process 'whereby knowledge is created through the transformation of experience'.

Embodied learning

Embodied learning is generally defined as the connection between bodily movement and cognitive ability; in other words, the relationship between mind and body within a learning context. Elaborating further, Munro (2018) defines embodied learning as the purposeful use and recognition of 'multimodal body-mind activities and strategies to facilitate shifts in perspectives, perceptions, paradigms, behaviour and actions'. Like Kolb's definition of experiential learning, embodied learning is also seen as being transformative, both in terms of knowledge and an understanding of self.

Play, within a creative arts context, is seen as being integral to the process of embodied learning and as Becker (2009) suggests, the deep, bodily immersion into the subject matter with 'the heart . . . the mind, and the spirit of play . . . will more likely come to grasp it at its core than those who rely on information, quantification, or objectification' (Becker, 2009: 59).

Reflective learning

Boyd and Fales define reflective learning as 'the process of internally examining and exploring an issue of concern, triggered by an experience, which creates and clarifies meaning in terms of self, and which results in a changed conceptual perspective' (1983: 99). The process of reflection, in the sense of an activity in which 'people recapture their experience, think about it, mull it over and evaluate it' (Boud et al., 1985: 33), can be seen as being integral to the process of experiential and embodied learning.

Reflexive learning

Reflexive learning is seen as a process of learning in which there is an active exploration of experience with the aim of becoming more self-aware, self-critical and open minded. It is a process of self-evaluation and revaluation, a reflexive loop as new information leads to new learning and an ongoing development of personal insight. Clearly, there are links between reflective and reflexive learning, the nuanced difference being that whilst reflection concerns insight and awareness, reflexivity can be thought of as a more active process of 'finding strategies to question our own attitudes, thought processes, values, assumptions, prejudices and habitual actions, to strive to understand our complex roles in relation to others' (Bolton & Delderfield, 2018: 13).

Other terms related to this discussion include *felt sense, flow* and *tacit knowing*, all of which are fundamental aspects of the learning processes as defined earlier.

A theory of being and doing: the role of experiential learning

> Tell me, and I will forget. Show me, and I may remember. Involve me, and I will understand.
>
> (Confucius 450 BC)

As highlighted by the preceding well-known dictum from Confucius, there is something of a classical, epistemological provenance to the concept of experiential learning. Certainly, the concept of learning through doing is not new, as further underlined by Aristotle in 350 BC, who said that – 'for the things we have to learn before we can do them, we learn by doing them'. As stated, the core ethos of child-centred play therapy (CCPT) places an emphasis more on *being* rather than *doing*, in that it is relational and process orientated, and whilst the aims, goals and outcomes of the work are clearly of great importance, it is recognised that these can best be achieved through a child-led process in which the child can experience a sense of control, autonomy and self-efficacy within the core, relational and attitudinal Rogerian conditions that underpin the theory and practice of CCPT. My premise within this chapter, as something of a counterpoint to the aforementioned, is that play therapy training is as much, if not more, about doing rather than being, or at best a complementary interplay between the two. Of course, in terms of experiential learning, the being/doing dichotomy is rather disingenuous, in that they are both intrinsically linked and are both key, interrelational aspects of the learning process, in that the *doing* of play therapy training, promoting self-awareness and personal insight, facilitates the *being* of clinical practice.

Moving forward in history, a rather more contemporary theory of experiential learning was established by Kolb (1984), a model that was (arguably) informed by the approaches of psychologists such as Jean Piaget (1953), Kurt Lewin (1935) and the aforementioned John Dewey. Kolb's very influential model (Figure 2.1), although critiqued, is widely seen as being synonymous with the theory of experiential learning, and is based on the premise that people learn through a four-stage cycle of *concrete experience (feeling), reflective observation (watching)*, abstract *conceptualisation (thinking)* and *active experimentation (doing)*. Within this model, effective learning is said to take place when the learner progresses through this cycle, entering the process at any stage. Allied to this learning cycle, Kolb also identified four distinct learning styles, which he summarised as *diverging (feel and watch), assimilating (think and watch), converging (think and do)* and *accommodating (feel and do)*. Within his theory, Kolb proposed that people have a tendency to fit within one of these four distinct styles, which will inform and impact upon their learning process. As Kolb describes:

Experiential learning is a process of constructing knowledge that involves creative tension among the four learning modes that are responsive to contextual demands. This process is portrayed as an idealized learning cycle or spiral where the learner 'touches all bases' – experiencing, reflecting, thinking, and acting – in a recursive process that is responsive to the learning situation and what is being learned.

(Kolb & Kolb 2005: 194)

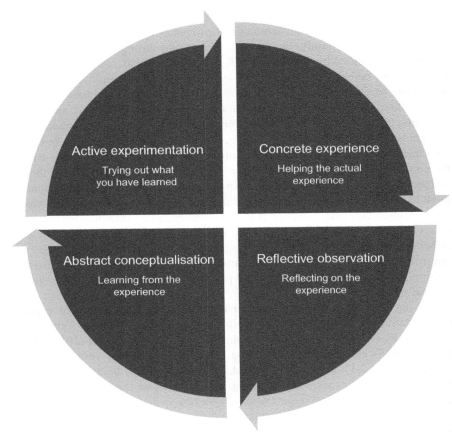

Figure 2.1 Kolb's Learning Cycle (1984)

The development of self-awareness and personal insight through reflective practice are key components of experiential learning, and applying the principles of Kolb's model to play therapy training, the trainee's learning is viewed both as a cognitive and an emotional, affective experience. As Kolb would say, it is a transformational process with new knowledge and awareness being generated as a result of new experiences, and so on through the cycle. This links to the principles of reflexive learning and is, I would suggest, a process integral to therapeutic training; a continual revaluation and integration of self-awareness and personal insight.

In a reappraisal/critique of Kolb's Experiential Learning Theory, Schenk and Cruikshank's (2014) model of Co-Constructed Developmental Teaching Theory (CDTT) proposes a biologically driven model of teaching and learning, in the light of emerging evidence from neuroscience. The CDTT model looks to conceptualise experiential learning within a sequential, neuroscientific structure, framing the teaching session within a set sequence i.e. *activity, direct de-briefing, reflective pausing, bridge-building* and *assimilation* and suggests that it is a model that could be applied in a variety of educational contexts. As they state:

> Experiential learning is powerful. However, we need to better inform ourselves about the mind–brain processes that affect experiential learning. When one understands why something works and can articulate that, it can be replicated in other contexts. In turn, this facilitates the potential application, not only in experiential education but also in other fields of learning.
>
> (2014: 18)

So, while Kolb's model has remained ubiquitous throughout Experiential Learning Theory, it is important that this is integrated into new models of learning, incorporating new and emerging evidence-based theory and research, especially within a neuroscientific context. As Schenk and Cruikshank suggest, there is a clear need for a new model of experiential learning that is 'grounded in current neuroscience research and able to facilitate predictable learning, yet adaptable as new understandings emerge' (2014: 18).

Within this context of emerging neuroscience and linked to the experiential learning principle of *doing*, research by Oppezzo and Schwartz (2014) suggests that walking i.e. active movement, increases creative ideation by an average of 60%, in comparison to those who remained sitting. The researchers hypothesised that the activity of walking may link to the process of associative memory, relaxing memory suppression and increasing associative ideation. Neurologically, this may link with aspects of 'down regulation' and the activation of less cognitively orientated 'flexibility pathways' (Baas et al., 2008). This links with Dietrich's (2006) notion of 'transient hypofrontality' and the suggestion that during physical movement the brain's neural resources are 'down-regulated' in order to direct bodily motion. The subsequent minimisation of activity within the prefrontal cortex allows a process of spontaneous creativity and ideation to emerge.

It may be something of a conceptual leap, but the aforementioned research might suggest that experiential learning that involves physical movement, play, action and embodied engagement can facilitate a neurological process of spontaneous, creative ideation, allowing a connection or flow between the theoretical, academic nature of the subject matter being taught and the more somatic, felt response to the memories, feelings and implicit associations that might emerge during the course of the experiential session. In this sense, it could be suggested that cognition is motion sensitive, connecting mind and body, thought and action.

Associated with the notion of embodied engagement, is Csikszentmihalyi's concept of 'flow' (Csikszentmihalyi & LeFevre 1989), which has often been linked to engagement in a task and which could also be applied to the experiential learning process. The concept of 'flow' can be characterised by the complete absorption in a task, activity or process, a melding together of action and consciousness. It is a concept often linked to physical activity, for example walking as discussed earlier and also running, but I would suggest that the deep immersion into an experiential learning activity, a process that involves the creative imagination, an interplay between the conscious and unconscious and a high level of emotional/affective engagement, can also evoke something of a flow state, linked perhaps to the dissociative process of reverie; that dreamy state of fanciful musing that can be such an important aspect of the play therapy experience. Akey (2006) suggests that being in a state of flow is indicative of a positive engagement in learning and certainly from my own experience, play therapy trainees have often described an intense and absorbed, focussed concentration on the experience of the present moment when engaged in experiential learning.

Experiential learning within play therapy teaching

As I have spoken about previously (Le Vay, 2022), acts of childhood remembrance are a key part of what it means to be a therapist working with troubled children, the therapy room playing host to those surprise visitors from our past, the countertransference stowaways, who have snuck aboard for the journey, only to appear when least expected. Perhaps we can also think of experiential learning in a similar way, in that it is a process that will inevitably involve a revisiting of the past and those early embodied experiences, non-verbally encoded, captured, within time and space. Michelson (1998) suggests that, as a function of memory, experiential learning could be understood as an act of 're-membering'.

> I want to make the case that experience is itself located in the body as well as in the social and material locations that bodies invariably occupy, and ask what a theory of experiential learning might look like that re-members body and mind . . . the body does not just hold the raw material for learning, but is itself a site of experiential learning.
>
> (Michelson, 1998: 218)

As well as my own learning experiences, there have been many times within my experience as a play therapy trainer when trainees have, in the process of an immersive experiential activity, shared profound moments of personal revelation, triggered by something in the creative process that has brought together past and present, something held both in mind and body; an unexpected jolt of self-awareness or realisation, a sudden previously unbeknown connection or association, a physical sensation of embodied remembrance, sometimes accompanied by tears, anger, surprise or joy. It might be a moment of sandplay, the symbolic significance of a particular object or image or a perhaps a sequence of movement. As Michelson (1998) suggests, experiential learning is sited within the self of the trainee, located within the realm of their lived experience, the hope being that there is an association, linkage or connection between the theory and the trainee's felt response to the theory, held within both body and mind. In this sense, the learning is in being able to *feel* the theory, as much as it is in being able to *know* it.

The notion of *felt sense* is important when considering the embodied process of experiential learning. The philosopher Eugene Gendlin, who first coined the term, describes it as follows:

A felt sense is not a mental experience but a physical one. *Physical.* A bodily awareness of a situation or person or event. An internal aura that encompasses everything you feel and know about the given subject at a given time – encompasses it and communicates it to you all at once rather than detail by detail. Think of it as a taste, if you like, or a great musical chord that makes you feel a powerful impact, a big round unclear feeling. A felt sense doesn't come to you in the form of thoughts or words or other separate units, but as a single (though often puzzling and very complex) bodily feeling.

(1981: 32–33)

Felt sense then, as Gendlin (1981) also rather nicely puts it, can be thought of as the soft underbelly of thought. We can think of it as emerging from a bodily, felt sensation, perhaps in the chest, stomach, throat or sometimes in the bodily extremities; legs, arms, hands or feet. Felt sense is not separate from thought, but sits, like tacit knowledge, on the edge of awareness, part of the same constellation of experience, even if the wider pattern and meaning is not immediately clear or recognisable. Often unclear, unsaid and unknown, it is an implicit awareness embedded in the body and beyond words. So, whilst unspoken and unremembered, felt sense can be thought of as something that sits within the liminal zone of our awareness, the threshold between the unconscious and conscious. Like the ebb and flow of tidal waters, that magical phenomenon of celestial shift, there is ever within felt sense the suggestive potential for movement, a crossing from one state to the another, and in this sense, it is a transitional, transformational experience. Felt sense is also, of course, integral to the relational experience of child-centred play therapy, part of the attuned process between therapist and child, in the sense that our own felt, embodied responses might be an important communication in relation to the child's experience of their own internal world.

Experiential learning draws deeply upon this rich wellspring of unremembered experience. Human experience can often be something of a battle between integration and separation; association and dissociation. As we know from working with children who have experienced overwhelming distress, there is a natural protective proclivity towards polarisation, or splitting, as we might think of it in terms of defence mechanisms, and just as within play therapy in which we aim to facilitate a process of integration – to untangle the knotted threads of feeling, thought and experience – as therapists we also need to untangle our own knotted past. Experiential learning and playful pedagogy are, I would suggest, critical, integral parts of this process. As discussed in Chapter 1, we all invariably carry our own, complex experiences of early, unmet need within us into our work, part of our pathway into training, and it is important that there is a methodology of reflective teaching and learning that can draw upon this rich resource, that taps into our felt sense and helps to facilitate meaningful, emotional and personal connections between theory and practice.

Jordi (2011), as an educator, spoke of his unease about a reliance on cognition and analysis to evoke meaning within learning, and highlights the need to develop more subtle, methodologies and tools of reflective, educational practice. As Jordi states, if we can

> conceptually engage with the complex intricacy of experiential learning with precision, then we can develop reflective practices that seek to facilitate an integration of the range of implicit and cognitive elements of our conscious experiencing. By identifying and engaging with elements that are characteristic of the integrative and meaning-making journey of experiential learning, I propose that we can develop a more expansive concept and practice of reflection.
>
> (2011: 195)

In simple terms, it is reasonable to assume that everyone learns from experience, but as Kuk and Holst (2018) suggest, 'it is one thing to link experience and learning, it is another to connect it to education' (2018: 155). When facilitating a session or lecture on a given subject, be it trauma, attachment, grief and loss or whatever the specific demands of the module in hand might be, I would ask myself the question; how can I embed the theory of this teaching into some sense of felt experience? How can the theory be brought to life? Often, the answer to this question is located somewhere within my own implicit memory; my own semi-conscious recollections of experiential learning that I had been a part of when I had been training to become a therapist i.e. learning experiences that had become in some way encoded within a felt, embodied memory; part sensory, part affective and part cognitive. For example, I remember a session as a trainee when we were asked to create a 'play genogram', using objects that symbolised different members of my family, including myself. I recall experiencing a profound response to the activity, both in a felt, affective way – a bodily response – and also in a more cognitive, intellectual way. It was an experiential activity that connected both mind and body, thought and feeling. Similarly, when training in dramatherapy, I recall powerful, poignant moments of group process in which we used role-play and dramatic enactment to explore and replay key moments from my early childhood. These moments in my own training, having been held so deeply on an affective level, have provided a valuable resource for my own teaching.

But also, experiential learning needs to sit within the learning aims and outcomes of a given session or module, so that there is a clear rationale around the use of a specific experiential activity and how this might fit in within the wider educational context of the teaching. There is a parallel here with clinical practice, in that the therapist, within the framework of child-centred play therapy practice, needs to be clear about the rationale for introducing a directed activity that will meaningfully connect with the child and enhance their therapeutic process, whilst also meeting the aims of the work. The challenge here then is about creating educational, learning experiences that are both relevant and meaningful, in that they both meet specific learning objectives and are appropriate to the learning style of the trainee(s).

Playful pedagogy: the role of play within experiential learning

As discussed, experiential learning, especially within the context of play therapy training, is key in enabling trainees to develop their capacity for reflective practice. It can help in the development of self-awareness and personal insight and through a process of embodied learning, facilitate an integrated, intuitive approach to education, to connect theory and practice within a personal context, and ultimately enable trainees to become more attuned, reflexive play therapists. Whilst the notion of experiential learning is not new, as we have heard from the likes of Confucius and Aristotle, the role of play within higher education has not been widely researched. Looking more broadly across the range of higher education and beyond that of just play therapy training, the more traditional, established convention of formalised, lecture-based practice tends to be the norm. It seems something of a shame that post-secondary, tertiary education has rather neglected the value of play within learning and the potential of a playful pedagogy. Indeed, Robinson (2011) went as so far as to suggest that the exclusion of play within tertiary learning is one of the great tragedies in education. Even within primary education, where one might think it would be enshrined in teaching practice, it could be argued that the role of play has been somewhat eroded, with an ever-increasing emphasis being placed on assessment, testing and government-imposed targets. Education is a serious endeavour, no doubt, but there is room I would argue for creative engagement and a process that honours the very fundamental role of play and playfulness within human learning.

Research by Forbes (2021) examined the role and process of play within higher education, from which the following key themes emerged: 1) play is underutilised and devalued in higher education, 2) play cultivates relational safety, 3) play removes barriers to learning, 4) play awakened students' positive affect and motivation, and 5) play ignited an open and engaged learning stance to enhance learning. As Forbes concluded,

> the results from this study provide additional legitimacy for play in learning as a substantial pedagogical approach in higher education. The results indicate that through play, students are better able to face the rigor of, and be more motivated to take risks and engage with, the material they are learning.

(2021: 70)

In summary, Forbes found that the introduction of play into the teaching reduced trainees' feelings of stress, fear and anxiety, facilitated a process of vulnerable engagement and enabled them to feel more connected to the teaching content. This suggests that the inclusion of play within higher education can play a significant, valuable role in enhancing the learning process, facilitating a much richer, deeper and connected experience of learning than if the teaching relied purely on the more conventional, standardised methods of delivery.

Ayling (2012) argued the potential value of play and play-based methods of teaching within social work training, especially in the context of teaching communication skills for direct work with children and young people, an integral aspect of the social work role. Whilst clearly a different role to that of CCPT, there are parallels and as Ayling points out, the inclusion of play in the teaching process of trainees who will be involved in direct work with children is in line with Ward's 'matching principle' (cited in Lefevre et al., 2008: 170) in which there is a congruence between the method of teaching delivery and the nature and style of the clinical process. This matching principle is an important, integral aspect of play therapy training, in that trainees have repeated opportunities to experience and engage in the therapeutic processes, approaches and, where relevant, specific activities that they will be using themselves to engage therapeutically with children.

For example, there have been many times as a trainee that I have completed a play genogram, as mentioned earlier, as an experiential learning activity. Each time is different; a symbolic, projective exploration of familial relationships at a specific moment in time. Just as one cannot step in the same river twice, the constant flow of thoughts, feelings and associations will forever bring with it new connections, meanings and insight, and with it an awareness of emotional triggers and areas of vulnerability. Before engaging a child in such a process, it is important that we have experienced this process ourselves so that we can be aware of the potential feelings that such an activity can evoke and be more empathic and congruent in the moment.

Ayling also highlights the potential benefits that play-based teaching can have for educators in meeting the varied range of peoples' differing learning needs and styles, as highlighted earlier within Kolb's model of experiential learning. Some trainees might be kinesthetic learners, others more auditory or visual. Importantly, within the context of experiential, play-based learning, Ayling also emphasises the need for a safe and contained learning environment with very clear expectations and agreements around confidentiality, respect and self-disclosure. As discussed earlier, experiential learning is likely to evoke often intense emotional responses and a degree of anxiety within trainees not familiar with this approach to learning, and in this sense, it is important to facilitate a structure of delivery that allows sufficient time and space for processing and emotional debriefing.

Structuring an experiential teaching session

To illustrate a process of experiential teaching and make links to the various processes described in this chapter, I will summarise an example of an experiential teaching session from my own experience. I would add, though, that experiential teaching is a flexible, adaptable process that needs to meet the differing needs of trainees at different points in their learning experience, at any given time. My experience of training has been that each group I have worked has been very different, and in this sense the delivery of experiential sessions needs to be carefully considered, be reactive and responsive, and be sensitively aware to the various needs of the group. The following example is of one experiential session in a moment of time and whilst it is a session that I facilitated many times, it will have changed and evolved.

Module topic

Working with trauma

Intended learning outcomes

- Overview of the neurological impact of developmental trauma.
- A basic understanding of physiological response to fear/trauma.
- Clinical play therapy implications for working with trauma.

Experiential exercise session plan

- Instruct group to each take a balloon, blow it up and hold it inflated without tying a knot.
- Each group member then takes a pin in their other hand.
- Instruct the group to stand in a circle, turning so that they are facing the back of the person in front.
- Instruct the group to gently hold the balloon against the back of the neck of the person in front of them and to hold up the pin in their other hand.
- **Do not allow anyone to burst their balloon**.
- After holding this position for a few seconds, instruct the group to lower their hand with the pin and to gently let the air out of their balloon.
- Put down the pins and the balloons.

Reflection/processing

- What was your immediate felt, physiological experience?
- What sensations did you notice within your body?
- Where in your body were these sensations located?
- What did you want to do?
- What were you feeling?
- What were you thinking?
- What was your relational experience?

Closure: Physical closure/shake down.
Discussion/feedback: Links to module topic.

Rationale

The rationale behind this experiential exercise was to safely introduce the trainees to the concept of developmental trauma through a process of initially *feeling* the module topic, prior to *thinking* about it. In this sense, the aim was to 'bring the material to life', which is often the way in which I might introduce the reason for an experiential exercise of this nature. To mirror the hierarchical, developmental nature of the brain, the exercise was structured to move in a bottom-up, sequential direction from a physiological, embodied experience to feeling and finally to thinking. In terms of processing the group's experience of the exercise, this was again done sequentially i.e. experience, feeling and thinking.

Processing

The preceding exercise was introduced at the very start of the teaching session, with little initial explanation or contextualising, beyond the fact that the group were aware of the module topic being addressed. Invariably, this experiential activity evoked some strong responses and considerable time was given to the group's feedback and reflections. In relation to the immediate embodied affective response, trainees talked about being aware of a raised heart rate, a shortness/holding of breath, a tightness in stomach/chest and a feeling of clamminess. Linking these somatic responses to *doing*, some shared the feeling of wanting to withdraw from the exercise (flight) and some questioned whether they could refuse to engage or follow my instructions (fight). Others reported feeling somewhat blank or being distracted by unconnected thoughts (freeze/dissociation).

In relation to feelings, trainees reported variously feeling anxious, nervous, apprehensive and excited. The relational context of the activity raised a lot of feelings e.g. anxiety about causing distress to the other person and what it was like to potentially have someone do something distressing to them. This was further explored within the context of relational, developmental trauma and links made to children's experience.

In relation to thinking, I began by asking the group to consider why we had engaged in this experiential activity. The group then began to make links between the module topic of trauma and their own responses during the exercise. They were able to reflect cognitively upon the experience e.g. what was happening within the brain, which areas were being activated within themselves at different times and how this linked to the specific function of the brain within a hierarchical, triune neurological model. Trainees reported a process of rationalising the experience, reassuring themselves of the lecture context, my role as lecturer, and the knowledge that no harm would take place. In this sense, there was a cognitive, 'wrapping around' of the limbic system, in an attempt to intellectualise and make sense of the experience and thereby managing/reducing any anxiety. After a physical warm-down 'debriefing' activity, we moved into the theory stage of the session, exploring the nature and impact of developmental trauma, the impact upon children and implications for therapeutic practice. Throughout this stage of the lecture, we often made links back to the earlier experiential exercise, linking the theory to their felt experience.

The sequential structure of the session is important, especially within the concept of working with trauma, in the sense of a process that mirrors the hierarchical model of brain development. I would suggest that were the session to be run the other way around i.e. to begin with the theory and then progress onto the experiential activity, the impact and the learning would not be as great. However, it is interesting to note that whilst this and most other experiential teaching sessions would be structured in this bottom-up, sequential manner, this was not an approach that I initially planned with any concrete rationale or reasoning. Rather, it just intuitively felt like the right structure; to begin with the feelings and then move into the theory and thinking. Latterly, I have been able to frame this more clearly within a neuro-sequential model of experiential learning, a process in which the theory becomes embedded within the trainee's felt-sense and both remembered and recalled on a somatic, embodied level. In this sense, it truly does become a process of bringing the theory to life, where it can be both felt and known.

A note of caution

It is important to state that the issues of safety and emotional containment were thought about very carefully at all stages of this experiential exercise. As I have talked about previously, people's pathway into therapy training may well have been informed by challenging life events, early unmet need and potential experiences of unresolved trauma. Trainees may or may not be aware of their personal, emotional triggers and in this sense, it is important that sufficient time is given to preparation, processing and debriefing. As trainee therapists, this also models the importance of safety and containment for the children that they will be working with.

At the beginning, I explained that we were going to be engaging in an activity that involved balloons and that they could choose to opt out, by either sitting out or leaving the room (many people have a strong, adverse reaction to balloons, and it is important to check this out). As with all experiential work, trainees were given the option to join in or not, ensuring that they had a sense of choice and control throughout the experience. At each stage, I was careful to check out how people were feeling, whether they felt happy to continue and whether anyone wanted to opt out. After the session, I facilitated a dramatherapy-based closure activity, specifically intended to shake out and discharge any affective, somatic responses. The timing of the activity within the programme was also important, in that I would only introduce an experiential activity of this nature when a group has been working together for some considerable time, so that they feel safe, familiar and comfortable working together in such a way. In this sense, just as in CCPT, the relational context of the process is important.

In thinking about trainee well-being and self-care, it is also important to acknowledge the role of personal therapy and (within some programmes) process groups, within play therapy training. Personal therapy, certainly for British Association of Play Therapists (BAPT) approved play therapy training in the UK, is a mandatory requirement, and provides an invaluable space for the processing of personal material that might be aroused during the process of experiential learning. As discussed, immersive learning of this nature will invariably, inevitably, connect trainees with early memories, associations and patterns of behaviour with an often surprising and startling intensity. Returning to the Confucius dictum of 'involve me and I will understand', the *doing* of experiential learning will evoke the *being* of the trainee, facilitating poignant moments of self-awareness and personal insight – those aspects of self-development that are such an integral part of training to become a therapist. As each experiential teaching session needs to be supported by a learning environment that feels safe, secure and contained, so the trainees overall learning experience throughout the duration of the programme needs to be emotionally held, to provide them with the secure base from which they can explore, play, experiment and take risks. Indeed, the programme holds an ethical duty of care towards the well-being of the trainee, just as the therapist has a duty of care towards the client.

Conclusion

Experiential learning can be creative, active and playful; a powerful and immersive process in which trainees develop not just a deep understanding of the subject matter but also a deep understanding of themselves. In training to become a play therapist, in which the use of self is the primary agent of change, the development of self-awareness and personal insight, as well as playful creativity, is a key, integral aspect of the learning process. As suggested, by learning through doing, they are also learning about being, a virtuous, reflexive experiential cycle, through which the trainee is continually gaining new awareness and insight into their own process. And as highlighted earlier, taking an active and involved role in their own educational process can also lead to increased levels of engagement and motivation, the personalised contextualisation of the process facilitating a more enhanced and meaningful learning experience. So, whilst not therapy, I would suggest that experiential learning of this nature is certainly therapeutic, being something of a 'learning laboratory' wherein trainees can experiment with new ways of being, explore new perspectives and gain insight into patterns of behaviour – developing an awareness of their learning edges and areas of both strength and vulnerability.

It is a shame, a lost opportunity, and perhaps as Robinson (2011) stated, a tragedy even, that creative approaches to education, including play and playfulness, have been so neglected. As said in the introduction to this chapter, my personal experience of secondary education was a chastening experience and was certainly one that did not allow any scope for creativity. Whilst academically I learned very little, it taught me a great deal about shame, failure and what it means to not feel good enough. Apart from sport, which was the one area in which I could succeed, there was little room for play. Instead it felt more a matter of survival and all in all it was a rather miserable experience, although I acknowledge that this could have been as much about my own story at the time as it was about the school's institutional failings.

But if secondary education was my road to perdition, then higher education was my road to redemption, and it was the role of experiential learning in particular that provided me with the language and opportunity to explore and make sense of some of the very difficult issues that had been hindering my progress. It is fair to say that it was no easy process, something of an emotional deep dive that proved to be both deeply challenging and deeply rewarding – high risk/high gain, as the saying goes. I cannot even say with any certainty that I undertook my therapy training with any conscious, overt plan to become a therapist. It was more an implicit recognition of something I needed to do, the process being so much more important than the result. Indeed, I recall very poignantly my dramatherapy interview with the programme convenor who deftly and sensitively guided our discussion towards my relationship with my father, as if she intuitively knew this was where the work was to be done. I am deeply indebted to her and the many other teachers and trainers across my various therapy trainings who played such a formative role in enabling me to (mostly) untangle the existential knots and frayed threads of my early years.

References

Akey, T. M. (2006). *School context, student attitudes and behavior, and academic achievement: An exploratory analysis.* MDRC. www.mdrc.org/sites/default/files/full_519.pdf.

Aristotle. *Nicomachean ethics* (c.334 BC – 330 BC).

Ayling, P. (2012). Learning through playing in higher education: Promoting play as a skill for social work students. *Social Work Education.* September, *31*(6), 764–777.

Baas, M., De Dreu, C. K. W., & Nijstad, B. A. (2008). A meta-analysis of 25 years of mood-creativity research: Hedonic tone, activation, or regulatory focus? *Psychological Bulletin*, *134*, 779–806.

Becker, C. (2009). *Thinking in place: Art, action and cultural production.* Boulder, CO: Paradigm.

Bolton, G., & Delderfield, R. (2018). *Reflective practice: Writing and professional development.* Thousand Oaks, CA: Sage Publications.

Boud, D., Keogh, R., & Walker, D. (1985). Promoting reflection in learning: A model. In D. Boud, R. Keogh, & D. Walker (Eds.), *Reflection: Turning experience into learning* (pp. 18–40). London, England: Kogan Page.

Boyd, E. M., & Fales, A. W. (1983). Reflective learning: Key to learning from experience. *Journal of Humanistic Psychology*, *23*(2), 99–117.

Csikszentmihalyi, M., & LeFevre, J. (1989). Optimal experience in work and leisure. *Journal of Personality and Social Psychology*, *56*(5), 815–822.

Dewey, J. (1916). *Democracy and education: An introduction to the philosophy of education.* New York: MacMillan.

Dewey, J. (1938). *Experience and education.* New York, NY: Kappa Delta Pi.

Dietrich, A. (2006). Transient hypofrontality as a mechanism for the psychological effects of exercise. *Psychiatry Research.* November 29, *145*(1), 79–83.

Fitzgerald, S. (1922). *The curious case of Benjamin Button. Colliers Magazine.* New York: Crowell-Collier Publishing.

Forbes, L. (2021). The process of play in learning in higher education: A phenomenological study. *Journal of Teaching and Learning*, *15*(1), 57–73.

Gendlin, E. T. (1981). *Focusing*. New York: Bantam.

Jordi, R. (2011). Reframing the concept of reflection: Consciousness, experiential learning, and reflective learning practices. *Adult Education Quarterly*, *61*(2), 181–197.

Kolb, A. Y., & Kolb, D. A. (2005). Learning styles and learning spaces: Enhancing experiential learning in higher education. *Academy of Management Learning & Education*, *4*, 193–212.

Kolb, D. A. (1984). *Experiential learning: Experience as the source of learning and development* (Vol. 1). Englewood Cliffs, NJ: Prentice-Hall.

Kuk, H.-S., & Holst, J. D. (2018). A dissection of experiential learning theory: Alternative approaches to reflection. *Adult Learning*, *29*(4), 150–157.

Lefevre, M., Tanner, K., & Luckock, B. (2008). Developing social work students' communication skills with children and young people: A model for the qualifying level curriculum. *Child and Family Social Work*, *13*(2), 166–176.

Le Vay, D. (2022). *Personal process in child centred play therapy*. London: Routledge.

Lewin, K. (1935). *A dynamic theory of personality*. New York: McGraw Hill.

Michelson, E. (1998). Re-membering: The return of the body to experiential learning. *Studies in Continuing Education*, *20*, 217–233.

Munro, M. (2018). Principles for embodied learning approaches. *South African Theatre Journal*, *31*(1).

Oppezzo, M., & Schwartz, D. L. (2014). Give your ideas some legs: The positive effect of walking on creative thinking. *Journal of Experimental Psychology: Learning, Memory, and Cognition*, *40*(4), 1142–1152.

Piaget, J. (1953). *Origins of intelligence in the child*. London: Routledge & Kegan Paul.

Robinson, K. (2011). *Out of our minds: Learning to be creative*. Minneapolis, MN: Capstone.

Schenk, J., & Cruikshank, J. (2014). Evolving kolb: Experiential education in the age of neuroscience. *Journal of Experiential Education*, 1–23. Sage.

Postcards from the playroom

For quite a few years I used to work as a therapist for young people in residential care; children who had been through multiple placements, foster families and adoptive families, but for whom things had not quite worked out. They had become the 'unplaceable children' for whom the only option was long-term residential care. The therapy room was on a site of three children's homes, and the young people would be brought over to their session by their link-worker, or sometimes make their own way over.

One boy, he must have been around 12 years old, took many weeks before he felt safe enough to spend the whole time in the session. He would stay for a few minutes, throw things around a bit and then leave. For some unbeknown reason, there was a sound system in the playroom and the boy would arrive with a CD of the heaviest drum and bass music you can imagine. He would put it on, turn the volume up to ten, and we would sit, unable to think or talk in this deafening musical maelstrom. I think he was waiting for me to tell him to turn it down or even off, which of course I never did. The windows rattled and shook with the vibrations and after each session I had to do a round of apologies to everyone else who worked in the building. They always knew when it was 4pm on a Wednesday afternoon. One session, as we sat bathed in air that crackled with sub-bass and heavy rap, the boy leaned across and turned down the sound system himself. That was the beginning of a tempestuous therapeutic relationship that lasted almost two years. I liked him very much, but he did enjoy giving me a hard time. One session, he turned up on his bike, insisted on riding it into the playroom and then spent the session literally running (or cycling) circles around me.

I remember one time it was winter and it had been snowing hard. At 4pm on that Wednesday the doorbell to the therapy building rang and I opened the door with my usual welcoming smile and friendly greeting. A massive snowball hit me right in the face. It was a great shot, but as I wiped the freezing snow and ice from my stinging eyes and saw him grinning in victorious delight, it was hard to hold onto a sense of empathy, let alone unconditional positive regard. They don't tell you when you are training how to deal with a huge snowball in the face.

Chapter 3

On not trusting the process

On not getting it right

During my time as a play therapy lecturer, there was a story I used to tell the students now and again about a young child I worked with many years ago; one of the many children that, as Lanyado (2003) says, we tend to carry around with us in our back pocket. She was 9 years old and had been placed voluntarily in care as a result of professional concerns around neglect and emotional abuse. The girl was one of several children and her mother was pregnant again, triggering her placement with a foster family. She was the only one of the children to be placed in care and was a very troubled, traumatised young girl; soiling, wetting, hoarding food and self-harming. She was also feisty and sharp-witted, grown up beyond her years, and certainly kept me on my toes.

In her sessions, week after week, she repeatedly played out a story through dramatic role play. In the story, she took on the role of a pregnant mother and I was given the role of her young son. Invariably, the mother would be about to give birth and we would have to dash to the hospital, always a race to get there in time. Following the baby's birth, we would return to the house, but whilst the mother and new-born baby were welcomed into the family home, I was told that there was no room for me and that I had to stay outside in the garden. From the cold, dark, rainy garden, I would give something of a mumbled commentary as I watched them through the window, welcoming home the new baby and getting on with family life. I would talk about how unfair it was that I was not allowed in, that the new baby was getting all the attention and that I was feeling upset and hurt. It felt like my mother did not want me, or had forgotten about me and I was no longer wanted in the family. This went on for some weeks, with a growing intensity, and whilst I clearly had a strong sense of what was being played out, I delayed making any interpretative reflections, thinking that I needed to hold my non-directive, child-centred stance and wait until the girl was ready to move the story on; that I needed to trust that the girl knew what she needed to do and would get there in her own time – that indeed I just needed to trust the process. Eventually, after many weeks of this, I grew frustrated and decided to make a more proactive, interpretive intervention.

DOI: 10.4324/9781003352563-3

Stepping out of role for a moment, I said something like,

You know what, I think I understand now. This story makes me think about how you might feel now – that you are left in foster care and your new baby sister goes home to live with mum. You feel left out – angry and hurt. It feels like mum doesn't want you.

The girl, turned to me, fixing me with her piercing blue eyes.

'At last, David, you big dumb-arse . . . you've got it!'

To be fair, I did feel something of a dumb-arse. I knew what the girl was communicating through her play, but I delayed making a reflective link to her real world, possibly because I was afraid that it would break the symbolic distance, or perhaps a reticence around being too interpretive. But the girl was clearly waiting for me to 'get it' and I missed important cues and opportunities within the therapeutic process, perhaps lacking confidence in my own intuitive sense or being too wedded to my non-directive position. Yes, she knew what she needed to do, but I stumbled in my capacity to be congruent, to use myself to connect with what the girl was needing to communicate; her need to be feel heard and understood. We all experience 'hits and misses' in our work as therapists, missteps we might call them, revisited in supervision, personal therapy or more often than not on our way home, the session ruefully replayed. But I remember all too clearly the lesson that this creative, resourceful child taught me that day – that one cannot and should not always trust the process.

Throughout my many years as a play therapist and lecturer, the phrase *trust the process* has seemingly become something of a mantra for the trainee and qualified therapist, a cliché even. It is a phrase often used to provide reassurance, for oneself or another; that in the face of uncertainty and challenge one can seek solace in the knowledge that there is an implicitly healing process in play and that, in a sense, the therapeutic process will look after itself. But it is also a phrase that I have increasingly begun to question. In this chapter then, I will provide a counter-argument to this position; to question whether it is in fact enough to trust the process and further, that in taking this position the therapist might absolve themselves of clinical responsibility and miss key issues around theory, evidenced-based practice and the active use of self to facilitate change within the therapeutic process.

Our role as play therapists is to enable children to feel heard and understood; to facilitate a process in which they can play out stories about often overwhelming experiences that all too often cannot be put into words. And our role is to listen. Children who have experienced relational trauma have been deprived of their voice, disempowered and silenced, and so as play therapists the most important thing we can do is to listen; with our minds, hearts and bodies, to respond with empathy and congruence to ensure that they truly feel heard. As Maya Angelou (1984) once suggested, there is no greater agony than having to bear an untold story. We also know that for children who have experienced trauma and abuse, their post-traumatic play might at times become stuck; looped, repetitive re-enactments of traumatic scenes that are more of a re-experiencing than a reintegration (Gil, 2017; Prichard, 2016). There can for children also be an agony in the telling of their stories, in the sense that it might feel unsafe and frightening; they may have tried to tell their story before and not been believed and more often than not disclosure is also a point of intense anxiety for children, demanding the need for trust and to feel safe and contained.

Returning to my example, the girl in question was using the creative process of dramatic play to very effectively communicate her experience. Over the weeks, something had become a little stuck, possibly connected to the traumatic nature of the story being played out and certainly within me and how I responded therapeutically to what was being communicated. Whilst we know that play is intrinsically healing and that play therapy is primarily a symbolic process, and that we do not necessarily need to link symbolic expression with experience for therapeutic change to occur, clearly in this case there was a need for a repositioning and a more active use of self to respond to the girl's communication, to both convey to her that she had been heard and understood and to facilitate the progression of the narrative. Sometimes we are afraid of getting it wrong, that our actions might have some detrimental impact upon the child or the therapeutic process, resulting in passivity or inaction. Sometimes we worry about doing harm, a feeling often sitting very powerfully within the countertransference when working with children who have experienced abuse and trauma and been so terribly harmed by the adults upon whom they have had to trust and depend. But sometimes also we need to take risks, and indeed there are risks in both action and inaction. I am confident that the child in question was not harmed by my missteps (frustrated perhaps) and we had been working together long enough for there to be a resilience in our relationship so that we could withstand these moments of rupture and repair. In fact, I was glad that this rather wonderful, resourceful girl felt able, with a hint of a smile and a mischievous glint in her eye, to call me a 'dumb-arse'; that she could feel emboldened and empowered to let me know that I needed to 'up my game', so to speak.

But if trusting the process means, as one online definition reads, letting go and having faith that things will eventually work out in their own time, then I would argue that this is not enough. Having faith in what? The theory? The play? The child? Ourselves? Yes, we can have faith in the process of play therapy, and so we should, but we also need to feel confident in our own sense of therapeutic agency and be mindful of not becoming disempowered through an over-adherence to a particular stance or position. Our work is informed by experience, but also by knowledge, theory, research, training, personal therapy and clinical supervision. Sometimes, within play therapy, the process becomes unhelpful, perhaps distorted or pulled out of shape by the unconscious dynamics of transference or countertransference, or those times when we might become triggered by the material. There might be moments of counter-dissociation (Valerio, 2017); embodied countertransference responses in which we might become cut off, defended or avoidant and experience blind spots or periods of unawareness that could impact upon the therapeutic process and prove unhelpful for the child. In these moments, it is not enough to trust that the therapeutic process will look after itself and to do so might prove detrimental.

Some thoughts on training

Of particular relevance to this discussion is the experience of play therapy trainees, for whom it could be suggested that the 'process' is not sufficiently known for them to place it in their trust, as they grapple with issues of newly acquired theory and skills and developing levels of self-awareness and personal reflection. Beginning trainees will often struggle with confidence and performance anxiety (Gibson et al., 2010; Skovholt & Rønnestad, 1992), for example in becoming pre-occupied or overly focussed on what they should be saying to the child, possibly missing important moments in what the child might actually be saying or communicating to them. Interestingly, research by Skovholt and Rønnestad that looked at the process of counsellors in training (1992) suggested that anxiety and a lack of confidence occurred in loops, recycling itself at significant stages in a professional's career, suggesting (perhaps not surprisingly) that we are all prone to periods of self-doubt and fears of incompetence (Cuschieri, 2016), which reach far beyond our initial training. Research by Brooks (2015) looking at the developmental process of play therapy trainees, highlighted issues around control, confidence and performance anxiety and the tension between holding onto a sense of control and letting the child lead the process. Significant within this research was a point in which the participants felt sufficiently confident enough to 'buy in' to the model of CCPT and with the support of clinical supervision felt more able to trust the play therapy process.

What may also help trainees to feel more confident in the therapeutic process is the sense of being anchored to strong theoretical and clinical foundations of practice. As Skovholt and Rønnestad suggest (2003), easily understood and applicable models, frameworks and systems of practice that can be absorbed quickly by the trainee can help to reduce feelings of anxiety. Clearly, within CCPT, there are tensions here between process and technique and the notion of *being* or *doing* and, of course, whilst being anchored provides a sense of safety and security it also, staying with the metaphor, can prevent movement. From my experience as a trainee, clinician and clinical supervisor, I know that one can become overly wedded to theory, especially in the early stages of training, resulting in the rather counterintuitive, paradoxical advice that I might sometimes give to students or supervisees to 'do less' or 'think less' and start to have faith in their own felt, intuitive responses to the child – to let go of the theory for a moment – in other words, to pull up anchor and allow the ship to drift with the current for a while. But I would argue that this is not the same as saying trust the process, the key being one's ability to recognise moments of stuckness, whether that is with the therapist or the child, and being able to proactively respond to these moments. At other times, the trainee might become too lost in process, caught up in therapeutic drift, requiring a need to reconnect with the theory and skills of CCPT and their own sense of agency. As therapists, we need tolerate moments of uncertainty, moments in which we might be unsure of the process and the direction or meaning of a child's play. The more confident we feel in our own knowledge, experience and theoretically informed practice, the more, I would suggest, we are able to tolerate uncertainty – to feel grounded and held in these challenging moments of not knowing.

Weighing anchor: frameworks, models and curious loops

Theoretical frameworks are integral to competent clinical practice and more often than not the challenge for therapists is being sufficiently attuned to the therapeutic process to know when to draw upon them. For example, Yasenik and Gardner's Play Therapy Dimensions Model (2017) provides a valuable decision-making framework to support and assist play therapists in how to position themselves in relation to the axes of directiveness and consciousness, supporting the therapist to make decisions about their level of immersion and interpretation. The model highlights four quadrants; active utilisation, open exploration, co-facilitation and non-intrusive responding – essentially providing a conceptual, organising framework that supports therapists in their decision-making around the use of self within the play therapy process. As a child-centred therapist, my 'comfort zone' is most often within the primarily non-directive quadrant of non-intrusive responding, working very much with the unconscious and emotionally/cognitively distanced process of symbolism and metaphor, particularly within the context of my work with children who have experienced acute developmental trauma. That said, I am also aware that being child-centred means responding to the needs of the child, from one moment to the next, and that this may require us to take other positions in terms of our use of self, degree of interpretation or level of directiveness. Going back to my earlier clinical example, by offering (albeit rather late) an interpretive reflection/response to the child's story I moved from a position of non-intrusive responding to that of co-facilitation, linking the child's play with the direct reality of her experience. Thus, having the support of robust models like the PTDM provides a theoretical framework wherein we can trust the process but also trust in *our* process as therapists and how/when/why we might make empowered, informed decisions to facilitate the therapeutic work, rather than a more passive faith (or hope) that the process will somehow take care of itself.

Figure 3.1 shows a play therapy model that conceptualises the play therapy process according to the two primary dimensions of directiveness and consciousness. The two dimensions intersect to form the four quadrants of active utilisation, open discussion and exploration, co-facilitation and non-intrusive responding

I have written elsewhere (Le Vay, 2019) about the improvisational play therapist, drawing upon the analogy of Keith Jarrett's seminal Köln Concert recording. In relation to trusting the process, one of the key aspects of this analogy is that Jarrett, famed for his capacity for solo piano jazz improvisation, was also an accomplished classical pianist. So, whilst the Köln Concert was a spontaneously

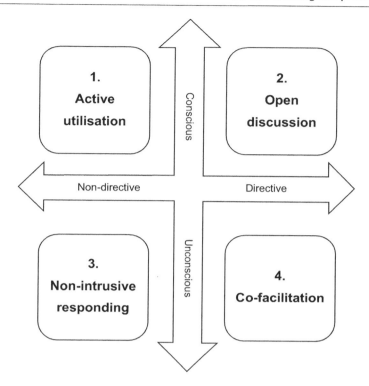

Figure 3.1 Play Therapy Dimensions Model
Source: Yasenik & Gardner, 2017

improvised piece of music, it was not without form or structure. Jarrett performed frequently and drew upon a variety of styles and techniques from which to respond to the moment, and a little like the Play Therapy Dimensions Model, he would have developed an internal framework, informed by theory and experience, from which he could scaffold, build and develop his musicality; a kind of internal repertoire from which he could draw.

Jarrett's playing was informed by a rich depth of patterned phrasing and intuitive characterisation honed over many years of experience and experimentation; a secure base from which he could explore, knowing he had a place to return to. This does not detract from the improvisational nature of Jarrett's playing, but simply provides parameters or a framework within which it can exist. This is, of course, analogous to the play therapy process, and that whilst we might indeed aspire to trust the process, it is a process informed by theory and experience as well as individual character and style. The theory underpins the practice, not in a way that restricts or inhibits the natural playfulness and curiosity of the therapist but rather provides the security of foundation and form. Being an accomplished classical pianist, it was Jarrett's very knowledge of the theory that allowed him to move away from it, just as the unconsciously competent play therapist is enabled to engage in playful improvisation within the playroom. As a musician and pianist myself, Jarrett's work has always been very close to my heart. His Köln Concert album accompanied the birth of my daughter, herself now an accomplished musician, so perhaps something of his creative, improvisational spirit has been internalised; osmotically absorbed into the family's musical narrative. Also, just to note, I am aware that I have been writing here about Jarrett's playing in the past tense. This is because a stroke in 2018 left him unable to use his left hand and, ultimately, no longer able to play the piano – or at least having to renegotiate his relationship with it. This again, as I have written about elsewhere, is something I can deeply relate to. Perhaps trusting the process also means being able to face up to one's limitations; to be honest about where our boundaries lie.

Knowing where our boundaries lie also suggests an awareness and confidence in our level of competence, again acknowledging the developmental learning continuum from novice play therapy trainee to experienced practitioner. Within this context, the Stages of Competency Model (Broadwell, 1969; Figure 3.2) is

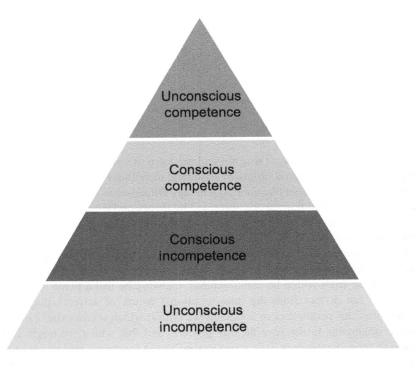

Figure 3.2 Stages of Competency Model
Source: Broadwell, 1969

helpful in providing a conceptual framework for this transition through different stages of learning, highlighting the two key areas of consciousness (awareness) and competence (skill). The model moves through the four stages of unconscious incompetence, conscious incompetence, conscious competence and unconscious competence. In the first stage (unconscious incompetence) the play therapy trainee is unaware of their lack of skill/knowledge and does not recognise this as a deficit or indeed as something they need to learn. The challenge here is for the trainee to recognise their own level of incompetence and the value of new skills and knowledge, before moving onto the next stage. Resistance might be a key factor here, as trainees struggle to 'let go' of aspects of their previous professional identity, within which they feel familiar, safe and secure. In the second stage (conscious incompetence), the trainee becomes aware of their lack of skill and recognises this as a deficit. This can be a particularly challenging period for the trainee as they become acutely aware of their own limitations regarding skill and knowledge. This is a key phase of learning and of being able to make 'mistakes', although paradoxically it can also be a time of acute anxiety around the fear of failure and of making mistakes, leading to paralysis and feelings of 'stuckness'. In the third stage (conscious competence), the trainee is aware of their skills and knowledge and has to work hard to consciously put this into practice. This might be a period in which trainees lean heavily into theory as new skills and knowledge are put into practice. In the final stage (unconscious competence), the experienced therapist has sufficient skill and knowledge for the work to be almost second nature and which, over time, has become internalised.

Whilst as trainees and qualified therapists we will understandably aspire to reach the point of unconscious competency, I would exercise a note of caution and suggest the addition of a fifth stage to Broadwell's Competency Model, that of 'complacent competence' – the point at which the learning curve perhaps begins to flatten out. As therapists we all need to ensure that we sustain, develop and enrich our practice through continuing professional development (CPD), clinical supervision and when appropriate, personal therapy. The learning never stops, and as I have said before, if a therapist ever feels they have no more to learn then it might be time for them to hang up their therapist hat. Similarly, we need to be mindful of issues of burnout and self-care (Topping, 2022) and the potential impact this can have upon our ongoing professional practice, and this plainly links to ethical frameworks and guidelines around the need to maintain professional competence within the profession.

Returning to the key discussion within this chapter, Broadwell's Competency Model is, I suggest, relevant to the question of how much one is able to trust the process. As we have seen, learning to become a play therapist is a developmental, transitionary process as we move through stages and degrees of competence and become more confident in our professional practice and developing identity as therapists. Clearly then, as we become more confident and competent, we become more able to trust the process – that our work is grounded in experience, knowledge and skill and self-awareness. Like Broadwell's model, we can equally see our capacity to trust the process as a developmental continuum. This has implications also for clinical supervision, which itself will move from being more educational and theory driven with the trainee, to something more reflective and process orientated with the more experienced therapist.

It could be suggested that to trust the process we need, as therapists, to be able to trust in ourselves; our responses, feelings, attitudes, behaviours and ultimately, our capacity to remain congruent, authentic and genuine in our therapeutic relationship with the child. In other words, to trust in our capacity to maintain the core conditions (Rogers, 1965) that provide the foundations of child-centred play therapy. Alongside being aware of the need to 'heal thyself', as explored in an earlier chapter, it can also be suggested that we need to 'know thyself'- as expressed through the well-known Greek aphorism, attributed to Plato, Socrates and Aeschylus, amongst others. Whether one can truly 'know thyself' is something of a contentious point, but central to this, within the context of play therapy, is the notion of reflexivity, which can be thought about as a process of internal attention – a form of self-dialogue in which we are able to reflect critically upon our thoughts, feelings, values and attitudes. Reflexivity, it can be argued, is a step further than reflection, a deeper, more intrapsychic, dynamic process in which there is cyclical movement between the 'inner' and 'outer' – a continual process of external awareness and internal integration. So rather than being simply a reflective understanding of our own process, reflexivity is more an active questioning of our underlying assumptions and responses, a kind of feedback loop, as we continually integrate and assimilate new information and awareness into our way of being – a much more critically dynamic and active process of self-reflection.

Staying with the image of loops, Schön and Argyris (1974) introduced the concept of single loops and double loops as conceptual models or frameworks for understanding reflective practice. Whereas single loop learning, as described by Gribbin et al. (2016), involves the 'creation and adoption of new action strategies in order to understand inner values' (2016: 6), the emphasis of double loop reflective learning is much more upon developing practice; an active process of questioning our values and assumptions with the aim of developing insight and awareness into what we do and why. This double loop model of reflective practice is more aligned to the concept of reflexivity and is, I would suggest, a necessary attitudinal condition for play therapists – an ongoing process of self-directed curiosity in terms of how we respond, react and relate within the context of our ongoing therapeutic learning and practice. The more we are able to question ourselves, the more we might aspire to the principle of 'knowing thyself' and the core conditions of congruence and authenticity and, ultimately, the more we might be able to trust the process. This links to the aforementioned notion of complacent competence, and having the self-awareness and personal insight to be aware of those times when our competence curve might be flattening out and our practice challenged by a variety of professional or personal circumstances.

But in grappling with the concept of what it means to be truly reflexive, rather than single or double loops, I find myself particularly taken with the Möbius Loop (Figure 3.3), which might be a more accurate depiction for exploring the notion

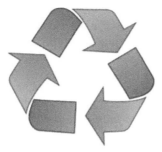

Figure 3.3 The Möbius Loop

of reflexivity and therapeutic congruence. As we know, a Möbius strip or loop is a strip of paper twisted in such a way that the distinction between 'inside' and 'outside' becomes indiscernible or indefinable. Whilst in one sense a representation of an abstract mathematical concept, a Möbius strip can also be simply constructed as a physical representation of this abstract concept – indeed, you could make one right now as you read this by taking a strip of paper, writing the word 'outside' on one side and the word 'inside' on the other. By giving the paper strip a twist before connecting the two ends, you will have created a Möbius strip, a strange physical shape with unusual properties. If you begin on the side where you have written 'outside' and follow with your finger, without lifting it from the paper, along the surface of the strip you will curiously find yourself arriving where you have written 'inside'. Continue, and you will find yourself back on the outside. The Möbius strip occupies a single plane; the inside and outside do not exist separately of each other, rather they flow – a continuous movement between the inner and outer with no barrier or boundary between them.

Within psychoanalytic literature (Wachtel, 2017), there has been some exploration of the Möbius strip as a metaphor for aspects of the unconscious process, but within the context of this discussion, I am choosing to use the image of the Möbius strip more as a metaphor for the process of therapeutic reflexivity, wherein there is a constant movement, a flow, from the internal to the external and back again as we experience, question, re-experience and re-question, an ongoing examination of our attitudes, feelings and responses. This is relevant both to the trainee play therapist, who is engaging in an ongoing personal process of developing self-awareness and personal insight, which will include the challenging of pre-conceived assumptions, implicit associations and unconscious bias, and also the experienced, practising therapist, engaging in ongoing clinical work and the intersubjective relationship between therapist and child. Similarly, we could write the words 'self' and 'other' on the two sides (or single side) of the Möbius strip, an image of the intersubjective process of overlap, or sometimes entanglement, or indeed the words 'conscious' and 'unconscious' as a way of depicting the flow between internal and external states of awareness. But however we might choose to play with the idea of the Möbius strip as a metaphor, the key existential quality of the image is of two sides existing as one; it is about movement, flow, tidal shifts, as the boundaries and barriers between inner and outer become increasingly fluid. The notion of intersubjectivity is key to this and as Stern states, 'our grasp of the external world, of course, is deeply influenced and informed by the internal one . . . this interaction is so continuous and complex that, in practice, the two worlds are completely entwined with one another' (2013: 638). The abstract and rather paradoxical qualities of the Möbius strip require something of a conceptual reimagining as we seek to consider both the intrasubjective and intersubjective nature of our experiential awareness, and therein our developing capacity for reflexivity. As Wachtel (2017) suggests,

> to take our insights the final steps toward genuine and lasting change in the patient's life, we need to walk along a new path. Conventionally, psychoanalytic thought has trod upon a path in which deep below the surface lies a hidden world, rendered invisible and inaccessible by that very surface. To expand our theoretical and therapeutic reach, we must also take a walk along that most unconventional surface of the Moebius strip, in which the continuous interweaving between inside and outside becomes apparent and the reciprocal dynamics of the psychic 'surface' and 'depths' are illuminated.
>
> (2017: 67)

As suggested earlier, the image of the Möbius strip as a metaphorical model for reflexivity, equally relates to the notion of congruence; the balance between felt internal experience and outward expression with the aim of a self-attuned matching or harmony between these states. Again, it is about the flow between the internal and external and in this sense, congruence could be viewed as an expression of reflexivity and vice versa. Reflexive practice demands an ongoing self-appraisal of our thoughts, feelings and behaviours, supporting us in maintaining the core attitudinal conditions that underpin the process of CCPT. The more reflexive and congruent we are able to be the more, I would suggest, that we are able to trust our own process and subsequently that of the child's.

But it is not, to paraphrase Erikson (1950), a simple case of trust versus mistrust. We live in a world that very much leans towards the binary: safe, fixed positions, a world of dichotomy and polarisation, one thing or another – social constructs that are more often than not framed as absolutes or unchanging opposites and which by definition can lead to splits, fragmentation and division. We can think of this within a societal frame, in terms of race, gender, class, politics, sport etc but also within the context of both the interpersonal and the intrapersonal – the relationship between self and other. I am drawn to the model of the Möbius strip because of its intrinsic fluidity, that there is not one side or the other but instead a sense of continuous movement and flow and I use it here essentially as a metaphor for the therapeutic process, whether that be in the context of clinical work, training, supervision or personal therapy. Perhaps it might be helpful in stimulating thought, debate or discussion around the theory and practice of play therapy and especially the dynamic process between child and therapist.

And so back to the beginning

I acknowledge that the title of this chapter is perhaps a little disingenuous, certainly provocative, but I hope in such a way that lends itself to discussion, to enable us to pause and reflect for a moment upon what we really mean by the term *trust the process* and to perhaps exercise a degree of caution as to how we use it, particularly within the context of training and clinical supervision. Of course, true to the ethos of CCTP, we should accept that play is a healing process and that being child led, we need to be able to trust the direction in which the child chooses to go; that consciously or otherwise, they know what they need to do. But to trust the process we need to be able to recognise and understand what that process is, that it is something informed and supported by experience, theory and supervision. As said in the introduction, it is not enough to assume that the process will somehow look after itself, that somehow it will come good in the end, because it might not, and we know from working with troubled, traumatised children that the process, both the child's and our own, is often a tangled, complex weave.

I am aware of many occasions in the past where I have possibly put too much trust in the process, become lost in it even, lost my sense of therapeutic agency, perhaps become too passive or indeed too active. Sometimes I may have worked with children for too long, or not long enough. Sometimes I may have been caught up too much in my own process – those beguiling narcissistic needs of the therapist to feel liked, needed or wanted. There have been times where I have clung too tightly to the theory, anchored and immobile, or let it go entirely, drifting without direction. There have been times, as I was so eloquently informed, that I have been a 'dumb-arse' and made mistakes or mis-steps in the work. Sometimes we get things wrong but most of the time we get things right and as trainees, therapists and supervisors we need to adhere to the principles of clinical responsibility and clinical governance. It is important that the mantra of *trust the process* does not become a default position or 'get out' clause; that it does not become a way of absolving ourselves from clinical accountability. Rather it needs to remain an active process of questioning and curiosity, supported by knowledge, theory and ongoing reflexive practice.

To return for a moment to the girl I talked about in the introduction to this chapter, I remember vividly the very challenging ending we had to our sessions, after working together for almost a year. The girl's foster placement 'broke down' (a rather odd expression within the terminology of the looked-after system) and she was placed in a residential children's home and I continued to work with her throughout this period as her social worker sought to find a new, longer-term placement. Her behaviour in the children's home was very challenging, including ongoing episodes of self-harm. One day she arrived for her session extremely angry and distressed and proceeded, as the expression goes, to trash the room – breaking things, upending furniture and tipping/squeezing out sand and paint. Much of this anger was directed at me, including her writing 'fuck off'' repeatedly on the white board. I was taken aback, surprised and shocked by the level of her rage, which she had never expressed before in her sessions, and had no sense or understanding of where this attack was coming from. The best I could do was to try to acknowledge the level of anger and distress she was expressing, to try and manage limits and keep us both safe, and it is fair to say that emotionally I felt rather battered and bruised when the session was over . . . as I am sure she did too.

Speaking later to the children's home, I learned that again the placement was 'breaking down' and it had been agreed for the girl to be moved at very short notice, within the next few days, to a specialist out of county placement, several hundred miles away. The girl had been told this prior to our session but no one had thought to inform myself, the therapist who had been working with her for the last year. So now I understood. Unbeknown to me, this had been our final session. I could understand her anger, her fury, her distress and most likely her profound sense of rejection and confusion, which interestingly – in a projective sense – were exactly the feelings that I experienced after the session. She would have understandably assumed that I knew about her move, and indeed that I was a part of it. She may even have thought that I had instigated it.

I tell this story as a poignant epilogue to this chapter, to emphasise that there is process both inside and outside the playroom and that sometimes it is something beyond our immediate control; that it is not something we can always trust. This young girl's trust in the process had been rather brutally shattered by the sudden premature ending of our sessions, as had mine, alongside her intense anxiety around her impending transition to a new placement. Systemic dynamics are important, as is communication within the professional network, so imperative in providing a holding, containing and secure foundation upon which the therapy can take place. We had both been profoundly let down by this system, just as she had felt let down by her family, perhaps sharing a sense of anger and betrayal. The door had once more been closed firmly in her face, leaving her standing again outside in the cold, dark garden looking in at the glowing lights and happy family within: the very place where I had once stood in that early session many months ago. Before she was taken to her new placement, I managed to negotiate one final ending session, with a hope of repairing some of the damage that had been done and to enable us to say goodbye. She arrived with her hairdryer, asked where she could plug it in and as she sat on the floor by the sandtray drying her hair she regaled me with the latest dramatic adventures of Hannah Montana, her idolised TV teen alter-ego. As Mark Twain (1897) said, 'truth is stranger than fiction, but it is because fiction is obliged to stick to possibilities; truth isn't'.

References

Angelou, M. (1984). *I know why the caged bird sings*. London: Virago.

Axline, V. (1987). *Play therapy*. London: Churchill Livingstone.

Broadwell, M. (1969). *Teaching for learning (XVI)*. wordsfitlyspoken.org. The Gospel Guardian. (accessed on 11th May 2018).

Brooks, T. P. (2015). *How therapy affects the counselor: Development through play therapy practice and supervision*. University of Tennessee.

Cuschieri, E. (2016). Can I really do this? An exploration into therapist self-doubt. In D. Le Vay & E. Cuschieri (Eds.), *Challenges in the theory and practice of play therapy*. Abingdon, UK: Routledge.

Erikson, E. H. (1950). *Childhood and society*. New York: Norton.

Gibson, D., Dollarhide, C., & Moss, J. (2010). Professional identity development: A grounded theory of transformational tasks of new counselors. *Counselor Education & Supervision*. September, *50*. Wiley/Blackwell, VA: ACA.

Gil, E. (2017). *Post traumatic play in children; what clinicians need to know*. New York: Guilford Press.

Gribbin, J., Aftab, M., Young, R., & Park, S. (2016). *Double-loop reflective practice as an approach to understanding knowledge and experience*. Proceedings of Design Research Society 2016 International Conference: Future – Focused Thinking, 8. Brighton, UK. pp. 3181–3198. ISSN 2398–3132.

Lanyado, M. (2003). *The presence of the therapist: Treating childhood trauma*. Abingdon, UK: Routledge.

Le Vay, D. (2019). The unplayable piano: From discord to harmony: Trauma, play therapy, and the power of the non-verbal. In A. Chesner & S. Lykou (Eds.), *Trauma in the creative and embodied therapies: When words are not enough* (pp. 33–44). Abingdon, UK: Routledge.

Prichard, N. (2016). Stuck in the dollhouse: A brain-based perspective of post-traumatic play. In D. Le Vay & E. Cuschieri (Eds.), *Challenges in the theory and practice of play therapy* (pp. 71–85). Abingdon, UK: Routledge.

Rogers, C. (1965). *Client-centred therapy*. Boston: Houghton Mifflin Company.

Schön, D., & Argyris, C. (1974). *Theory in practice: Increasing professional effectiveness*. San Francisco: Jossey-Bass Publishers.

Skovholt, T., & Rønnestad, M. (1992). Themes in therapist and counselor development. *Journal of Counseling and Development, 704*, 505–515. Wiley/Blackwell: ACA.

Skovholt, T., & Rønnestad, M. (2003). The journey of the counselor and therapist: Research findings and perspectives on professional development. *Journal of Career Development, 30*(1). New York: Sage Publications.

Stern, D. B. (2013). Field theory in psychoanalysis, part 2: Bionian field theory and contemporary interpersonal/relational psychoanalysis. *Psychoanalytic Dialogues, 23*, 630–645. https://doi.org/10.1080/10481885.2013.851548.

Topping, S. (2022). Self-care: Another important relationship. In D. Le Vay & E. Cuschieri (Eds.), *Personal process in child centred play therapy* (pp. 138–159). Abingdon, UK: Routledge.

Twain, M. (1897). *Following the equator*. Hartford, CT: American Publishing Company.

Valerio, P. (2017). *Introduction to countertransference in therapeutic practice: A myriad of mirrors*. Abingdon, UK: Routledge.

Wachtel, P. (2017). Psychoanalysis and the moebius strip: Re-examining the relation between the internal world and the world of daily experience. *Psychoanalytic Psychology, 34*(1), 58–68. APA.

Yasenik, L., & Gardner, K. (2017). *Play therapy dimensions model: A decision-making guide for integrative play therapists*. London: JKP.

Postcards from the playroom

I remember working with a boy who was very taken with the huge dressing up box that we had in the corner of the playroom. He particularly liked the very voluminous, colourful dresses that he dug out of the box with a barely supressed glee. He would use face paint to do his make-up and then promenade around the room in splendid grandeur. This was in the 1990s, long before the current transgender debate, and at a time when such behaviour was rather more pathologised within framework of gender dysphoria and even paraphilia.

Sometimes he would want me to wear a dress too, and we would sit, a very glamorous couple, and take tea together in the very fancy Victorian-esque tea house of his imagination. During one of these moments, a woman burst into the room, ignoring the 'session in progress' sign on the door. She did a classic double-take, raised an eye-brow and left with a very quizzical expression on her face. Such is the life of a play therapist. After the sessions he sometimes wanted us to walk back together, arm in arm and in full regalia, to the children's home where he lived. It took a bit of work to convince him that this would probably not really be appropriate.

I recall one particular session when the boy had found a dress that he especially liked and hauled it over his head, lost momentarily within a fantastic bustling flurry of lace and linen. With the dress finally on, he twirled around a few times and then, looking at me over his shoulder, asked in all earnestness, 'does my bum look big in this?' They don't tell you about this in training either.

How much this was about gender identification, I am not sure, and I don't think any kind of labelling was especially helpful. Having experienced early maternal deprivation, been very neglected and spent most of his life in care, I think he was simply finding ways to feel close to his mother, even be his mother. But in the end, it does not matter too much what I think, the important thing being that he felt free and able to be whoever he chose to be.

Chapter 4

Stormy weather

On not being good enough

Moderate or good, occasionally poor

As a young child, I was never sure whether my father loved me. I assumed not, having no evidence to suggest otherwise. But I did know that he didn't like me, which was somehow worse. To not feel loved somehow did not matter; love was an elusive, illusory, abstract thing, hard to quantify or understand. It was either there or it wasn't. But to not feel liked was raw and abrasive, it cut like a wound. It both numbed my edges and froze my core . . . as if there was nothing about me worth liking. As I have written about previously (Le Vay, 2022), my relationship with my father was complex, mostly governed by his often extreme mood swings, his emotional unpredictability and his brooding, intense depression that enveloped the family like dark, bitter treacle. His parenting strategy at times was nothing short of an emotional attack. He sought to shame, humiliate and demean.

There were exceptions of course; brief periods when the storm clouds lifted and he could be charismatic, engaging and playful, exciting in his manic exuberance and vibrant, infectious energy. But always conditional and on his terms. In time, as I got older, I came to understand this but as a child and young adolescent there was no sense to be made. Thankfully, I had the counterbalance of my mother's unconditional love and affection that smoothed some of the rough edges, but in relation to my father I was never good enough. It was (is) a powerful script, etched into my psyche; the words might smooth and fade away over time but will never quite be erased. I was not a good enough child. Not a good enough son. Not a good enough teenager. Not a good enough adult. All I wanted was his approval, but it never came. I remember telling him, in my mid-20s, that I had qualified as a social worker. I thought he might be proud. Instead, he just looked at me coldly and said, 'well . . . I think all social workers should be shot'.

After my father died, going through his papers with my family, we were surprised to find an unpublished, alternative version of his autobiography. In one section he gave an account of his many years of 'failed' psychoanalysis, which finally

DOI: 10.4324/9781003352563-4

led to a consultation with the esteemed paediatrician and psychoanalyst, Donald Winnicott. My father wrote of that meeting:

> Winnicott sat opposite me, put his hand over his eyes – not the usual form – and did more for me in an hour than anyone else in a year. He began by saying, 'you know, I had the feeling that you might be coming for me with a gun' – quite amazing intuition since this had been exactly my own visual imagining. He also told me that I had to be my own father, having denied (or been denied) a loving paternal relationship. That too was exactly right and no-one had ever said it before.
>
> (Le Vay, 1970: 120)

In a strange way, I feel deeply and personally indebted to Winnicott. Reaching out from the past, he has helped me understand something about my father; that he never felt good enough either, never felt loved or indeed liked by his own father. I finally felt a connection, a sense of mutual recognition, empathy even, that I had not felt before. Like Winnicott, I often felt that my father was 'coming for me with a gun', so to speak. But now I can understand why – that he had himself spent a lifetime trying to avoid being shot.

Thankfully, before he died, my father and I were, to an extent, able to make our peace, for which I am eternally grateful. He told my partner that he did love his children, but was just not able to tell us himself . . . that he did not know how. I wrote to him, telling him, amongst other things, that I had qualified as a therapist, flinching, ready to dodge the bullet. He wrote back to me – I am looking at his letter right now as I write this – which consists simply of two typed lines. He wrote, 'I have always been impressed by your capacity for love and patience and identification, which might, in other circumstances, have led to you becoming a priest. Short of that, being a therapist is what you may well have been put on earth for'. Was this a confession? Absolution? An apology? It might even have been approval.

Given the preceding, I have thought a lot about what it means to be good enough and about those times, as play therapists, when we might not be feeling good enough. Winnicott's (1953) writings on this subject have become embedded within play therapy discourse – the good enough therapist – alongside a child-centred theoretical framework that moves away from the position of therapist as expert and toward a more collaborative, constructivist stance that acknowledges our own stories, alongside those of the child. As play therapists we talk about 'conditions of worth' and those factors that impact upon a child's developing identity. We are working with children who are not feeling good enough, or who are perceived as so, through the very act of being referred for therapy. So, there are complex areas of entanglement between the child's and the therapist's process and the stories we tell about ourselves. Within this chapter, I aim to explore a little of this entanglement, the questions around therapist conditions of worth and the challenges and dilemmas for some around powerful internalised narratives of perfection and parental messages of expectation. This links closely to the discussion in Chapter 1, which explores the question of both conscious and unconscious motivations to train. I will draw upon Winnicott's (1953) concept of 'good enough' as the main theoretical basis for this chapter, due both to the seminal contribution his work has made to the profession of child psychotherapy, and partly also due to the somewhat vicarious personal association mentioned earlier. I will also draw upon clinical material, as a way of illustrating some of the potential parallel processes at play.

Smooth, occasionally rough, becoming variable

Knowing how and where to begin this chapter has been a considerable challenge; this is one of many attempts, and many beginnings. It is like trying to shine a light on something that almost by definition does not want to be seen; it recoils, retreats, under the unwelcome gaze, avoiding scrutiny at all costs. It is something that shuns observation, to the point that we doubt its very nature. Is it really there? And perhaps this is something to do with the very essence of what it means to not feel good enough, because to not feel good enough taps into deep-seated feelings of shame, humiliation and guilt – feelings that thrive in the half-light of our early years. Shame, in particular, is all pervasive. It seeps through the cracks of one's very being, coalescing into liquid pools of burning hurt that gather in the emotional folds, the nooks and crannies, of our sense of self, permeating through and into the very core of one's identity. An insidious ingress, an infusion of sorts; a stain on one's character, one might say. Shame lingers, like an unwelcome midnight guest at the end of a party, reluctant to be ushered out of the door into the cold dark of night. As Wright (2022) suggests, shame has the ability to lurk, hidden and undetected – but always there.

For as long as I can remember, I have striven to be good enough. In my rational mind, I know that I probably am; I have had a successful career, a loving family, good friends, but lodged deeply within the recesses of my emotional brain – and sometimes in my stomach – the not good enough voice has a habit of making itself heard. I recall once talking to a friend about her experience of organised religion, and of guilt in particular. She described it as like having a small explosive device implanted deep in her head, the small but frequent detonations a critical reminder of its presence, the harsh bang on wood of the judge's gavel. This is like the voice of the not good enough, and I would venture that it is a familiar voice to many therapists.

In the first chapter of this book, I explored some of the connections between our early, formative, childhood experiences and the desire, conscious or otherwise, to train as a play therapist and work with troubled children. Whilst cautious to generalise – our experiences are individual and unique – it would seem more often than not that the motivations to pursue a career as a child therapist is rooted in relational experiences of unmet need. I would not, though, necessarily frame this as a negative. Indeed, it is this very experience of unmet need that provides us with the inner drive, motivation and ability to be able to connect with children who themselves have experienced relational turmoil. The capacity as a therapist to be able to recognise and attune to the not good enough child comes, I would suggest, from a place of being able to recognise this within ourselves – a form of mutual recognition that is in itself the very basis of empathy and empathic connection.

The notion of 'good enough' has become enshrined into therapist lore, a legacy of the seminal work of the aforementioned Winnicott (1953), first introduced in his deeply influential paper *Transitional Objects and Transitional Phenomena – a Study of the First Not-Me Possession*. Here Winnicott writes:

> There is no possibility for an infant to proceed from the pleasure-principle to the reality principle or towards and beyond primary identification . . . unless there is a good enough mother. The good enough 'mother' (not necessarily the infant's own mother) is one who makes active adaptation to the infant's needs, an active adaptation that gradually lessens, according to the growing ability . . . to tolerate the results of frustration.
>
> (1953: 93–94)

Winnicott proposed that the 'good enough mother' starts out by adapting as much as possible to the infant's developing needs. The mother is responsive and devoted, sacrificing her own needs to fulfil those of her baby – to be present, receptive and empathically attuned at all times. The mother and baby are as one, the baby experiencing the mother as part of him or herself. Over time, as the baby develops, physically and cognitively, and begins to experience the external reality of its world, the 'necessary illusion' of the perfect mother is gradually replaced with the 'good enough' mother who allows the baby to begin to experience small amounts of frustration, to be able to tolerate not having its needs met at all times. This transitional, developmental shift from 'perfect' to 'good enough' stimulates and facilitates the baby's cognitive and emotional development and is the beginning of the infant's sense of becoming a distinct being; of a process of psychological separation and playful exploration. Winnicott argued that a too perfect mother would inhibit the infant's process of discovery and exploration – that the infant could become stuck or fixated with the fantasy that every need or desire will be immediately fulfilled. In this sense then, the mother's 'failure' to meet the child's every need is a critical part of individuation. As Winnicott suggests:

> A mother is neither good nor bad nor the product of illusion, but is a separate and independent entity: the good-enough mother . . . adapts less and less completely, gradually, according to the infant's growing ability to deal with her failure. Her failure to adapt to every need of the child helps them adapt to external realities.
>
> (1953: 89–97)

Of course, for good enough mother, we can think of good enough parent, in all its forms and roles and as a further extension, the good enough therapist. As discussed previously, those early, relational experiences of unmet need that might contribute to our motivations to train as therapists and work with troubled children can also connect with therapists' feelings of expectation, imperfection and failure. We might, as therapists, strive for perfection, but as Winnicott suggests, this might not be desirable and indeed, the core principle within CCPT of returning responsibility back to the child is part of the process of enabling the child to tolerate small experiences of frustration and from that, autonomy and mastery. Children in play therapy will seek approval and praise, to provoke those conditional patterns of relating with which they feel so familiar, the desire for the perfect therapist/parent perhaps. The core condition of unconditional acceptance means that whilst we may not be able to respond to all their external needs in the way that they want, we can help children develop their internal sense of self-worth – that they are indeed, good enough. Drawing on this parallel between parents and therapists, Cozolino (2004) suggests that as good enough therapists we can surrender, or in Winnicott's words, adapt, to our imperfections and failures, whilst still being able to facilitate a therapeutic relationship that leads to positive outcomes. We may well make mistakes, but as Cozolino rather nicely puts it, good therapists make good mistakes.

Within Winnicott's concept of good enough, the notion of parental 'failure' might also be seen as the making of 'good mistakes', small acts of unmet need that promote the infant's developmental growth and facilitate an experience of autonomy and individuation. Within this context, failure can be understood as a healthy part of the good enough parent just as, to continue the parallel, failure might be seen as a healthy part of the good enough therapist. I have been in personal therapy at various points during my career, and the idea of the perfect, omnipotent, omniscient therapist is rather terrifying and would probably reduce me to emotional shreds. I recall once working with a personal therapist who seemed to doze off at times in our session, engendering within me a rather devastating sense that I was boring her – that I was not worth listening to – and this triggered very early, childhood feelings of paternal rejection. After several weeks I plucked up the courage to challenge her about it and to tell her how she was making me feel. It was an awkward moment and I eventually decided to find a different therapist, but the experience actually left me feeling empowered; I took control and made a choice and was able to assert and prioritise my needs, not something I am generally very good at. So, in a strange way I was very grateful to the therapist for giving me what in the end felt like something of a personal gift – the power of self-agency and self-efficacy. I was rarely able to challenge my father.

There is both humility and humanity in failure. As therapists we understandably strive to defend ourselves from feelings of failure, feelings of not being good enough, punish ourselves for making perceived mistakes and protect ourselves from futility – perish the thought that our efforts as therapists might be ineffective. But it may be that failure, the making of mistakes and the act of being human, and therein occasionally vulnerable, can powerfully connect us to the children and families that we work with. As the psychologist Sachs (2020) suggested, clinical success can paradoxically hinge upon the capacity to acknowledge failure – 'because when we acknowledge our failure, we acknowledge our humanity, and when we have the patience and courage to experience *shared* failure, we acknowledge our *shared* humanity, which leaves us feeling a little less alone in the world' (Sachs, 2020).

Conversely, if we are to think about 'good enough' we also need to reflect upon what it means to be 'bad enough' (Abramovitch, 2021), both from the experience of the child and the therapist. Abramovitch talks about the importance of recognising (as well as acknowledging and accepting) when the therapeutic process has become 'bad enough' that it becomes necessary to instigate change and particularly, as Abramovitch writes, make those difficult decisions about ending. These moments can be challenging and complex. As Abramovitch suggests, it is easier to recognise a good enough situation than a bad enough one –

> being good enough typically means continuing what you are doing in a relaxed, wholesome manner. Being bad enough usually implies the need for painful and uncertain change. The danger of the bad enough situation is it becoming even worse. Whereas feeling good enough is experienced in the present, bad enough must consider both past, present and future in a complex algebra of emotions and expectations.
>
> (2021: 920)

As Abramovitch says, the feeling of not being good enough, or indeed of feeling 'bad enough' might on occasion demand difficult and painful decisions around how we work as therapists and during these periods, the support of personal therapy and clinical supervision can be critical. Part of acknowledging 'our humanity', as Sachs puts it, also means acknowledging the need for self-care and possibly even fitness to practice. We might need to reflect carefully upon the kind of work we undertake, our caseloads and the prioritisation of our own needs (not always a strong point for therapists). Life events will invariably knock us off course, challenging our capacity for resilience and robustness. Therapists are not invulnerable, and there is strength in being able to acknowledge this. I have personally been confronted with this experience when, in the face of a recent, challenging health diagnosis, I had to think carefully with my supervisor about my own fitness to practice and how I managed my clinical work in a way that felt safe and ethical, both in relation to myself and my clients.

Veering slowly, losing identity

Children who have experienced relational, developmental trauma and who have been referred to play therapy are more often than not having to manage profound feelings of shame, guilt and poor self-worth. Rather than the good enough parent, their experience has been of the 'bad enough parent', the parent who has not been able to adapt sufficiently enough to meet their basic needs. This brings us to Winnicott's (1965) notion of the false self, wherein the child who has not received good enough parenting, whether through parental anxiety, depression or more wilful acts of abuse or neglect, learns to suppress their natural, expressive spontaneity in order to comply with the parent's needs, wishes and feelings. In this sense the child directly experiences the external stress of the parent's world, the only remaining strategy being for the child to withhold and suppress their natural desires as a way of winning back, or regaining parental attention and/or affection. A false self is established when the expectations and needs of the 'other' become of overriding importance; opposing, contradicting or overlaying the sense of true self that lies at the heart of the child's being. In short, the child learns to be not good enough in order to maintain a good enough parent, their fragile psyche, the core self, something to be defended and protected.

It is suggested that the true/false self dichotomy is better understood as something of a continuum, that the false self, to one degree or another, is an adaptation that we all have to make to survive as social beings – the caretaker of the true self. But for children who have experienced acute, early relational trauma, the need to defend their fragile core identity is a matter of psychological survival and a significant contributory factor to the complex attachment patterns that as therapists we often find ourselves working with. These are children that have learned to hide in plain sight, who are continually striving to protect and defend themselves from psychological distress, although paradoxically I would suggest that these are also children desperate to be seen; children who want to be close but are afraid to be near.

Winnicott also said that 'it is a joy to be hidden and a disaster not to be found' (1965: 187) and therein lies the existential paradox, the inherent tension in our work as play therapists working with children who have such a profound need to be seen, to be heard and understood, whilst also seeking to protect their core, isolated self that lies at the heart of their fragile identity. As Pitt (2000) suggests, communication in itself is often experienced as an urgent game of hide and seek and, of course, this validates the importance of therapeutic play and the 'as if' quality of symbolism and metaphor and of engaging in the space beyond words. But there is a tension nonetheless, between compliance and authenticity, attack and defence, acceptance and denial. Winnicott also talks, somewhat counterintuitively, about the client's right not to communicate and as Pitt says, Winnicott's notion of an 'isolated and secret self along with his insistence upon the individual's right and need to resist the (therapists') interpretations create a puzzle for psychoanalysts, who are among those professionals sought out when life fails to feel satisfying' (2000: 66). As Winnicott himself puts it, the question is 'how to be isolated without having to be insulated?' (1965: 187).

And indeed, it can be quite a puzzle, as we seek to find ways to connect with the very emotionally defended child. It is not our job as play therapists to dismantle children's defences; these are important, necessary protective strategies that they have developed over many years, a delicate, psychological, proximal balancing act that allows the child to remain both 'connected to' and 'distanced from'. I have often thought about how psychologically exhausting it must be for children to have to continually walk this tightrope. But Winnicott's question is also one that many of us might be able to relate to; that like the children we work with, we also have to negotiate the tension between good enough and not good enough. Like some kind of osmotic, semi-permeable membrane, the defensive shields that we erect around ourselves allow for emotional transfer between inner and outer and vice versa. If my rather sketchy memory of school biology is correct, osmosis involves the transfer, or movement, of solute molecules from a stronger solution to a weaker solution – a direction that ultimately serves to equalise both sides of the dividing cell membrane. A rather laboured metaphor perhaps, but in a sense, this is what we might hope for as therapists, that the more fragile, weaker internal self is gradually fortified and strengthened through the therapeutic relationship, building feelings of self-esteem and self-worth.

As therapists, we are working with children who are defending themselves against feelings of not being good enough. It is, after all, what has brought them to therapy. As therapists, we are also working with our own feelings of not being good enough. It is, after all, what has brought us to therapy. I often reflect upon Winnicott's notion of good enough and the false self in relation to some of the adopted children that I work with, children who have by definition had very early, formative experiences of relational trauma, abuse, neglect and separation. These are children whose birth parents, often for very understandable reasons related to their own complex history, have not been able to adapt to their infant's needs. Indeed, it is often the infant that has had to adapt to their parents' needs and these are the children who may well have a developing sense of not being good enough.

The Queen's Gambit

I recently found myself playing chess with a 12-year-old boy, I will call him Andrew, who had been adopted at the age of 5. His background was one of domestic abuse, neglect and maternal drug and alcohol use, and he had several moves between foster placement before finally being adopted. He is a child with a fragile sense of self-worth, very emotionally defended and unable/unwilling to directly explore issues relating to his early years. Within his adoptive family, he manages well although sometimes experiences intrusive, distressing thoughts about death and dying, struggles with feelings of self-esteem and self-worth and finds it hard to sustain positive peer relationships.

In his early sessions, Andrew chose to play games on the whiteboard. Word games, puzzles, hangman, squares, mathematical challenges but most of all, endless games of noughts and crosses, or tic-tac-toe, as he called it. We would sit opposite each other, with the whiteboard resting on our knees, forming a bridge between us. He loved to strategise and work out all the possible permutations; game after game, session after session, week after week. In-between sessions he would play online, frustrated that he could never beat the tic-tac-toe computer. We were seriously competitive, but also seriously playful, and at times we laughed, joked and had fun together. But I found myself preoccupied with the familiar feelings of self-doubt; was this therapy? Is this good enough? Am I a good enough therapist? The sessions were being funded by the local authority, and I anxiously wondered how

I might justify playing noughts and crosses in the next review meeting. Reflecting upon this, I can see now that it was more about the playing than it was about the game. It was about building our relationship, finding a way to be together, feeling connected by the whiteboard, about laughter and humour and playful competitiveness. Yes, there is perhaps also something about the game; the turn-taking, the sequencing, the patterning – something that is structured, ordered and rule-bound. Often, I think the question with games is about how much they are the therapy and how much they are a defence against the therapy, I guess a bit of both. But the essence of noughts and crosses is about connection, both literally and relationally.

Then one week Andrew asked if we could play chess. He said there was something he wanted to talk about but found it very hard and that it would feel easier if we had something to do and were not looking at each other. Eye contact, within the context of shame, guilt or anxiety, can feel challenging, dangerous even, that in being 'seen' or 'known' there is the risk of rejection. The need to look away, the avoidance of the intrusive gaze of the 'other' might also be a protective strategy and, in the context of adoption, makes me think about the baby's experience of having to regulate affect, in the absence of the parents' capacity to do so.

Andrew is a good chess player and we both became engaged in the game, pausing at times for him to talk, if and when he so chose. As we played, he was able to say a little about how he had been getting upset recently thinking about death and dying, especially at night, and between the chess moves we dipped in and out of exploring his thoughts and feelings – his fears and anxieties, the possible patterns and triggers around these feelings and potential strategies he and his parents might use to help him manage when his distress became too much. I reflected briefly upon his early years with his birth family and his adoption and Andrew switched to a playful robotic voice, letting me know that this was too much and to not go there. Adoption is hard; children who have been adopted struggle with profound feelings of rejection, abandonment, of not being wanted, indeed of not feeling good enough – not feeling loved or liked. I wondered to myself about Andrew's fears around death and dying; the fragility of his core self perhaps indicative of a 'deadness' that he has to work hard to defend himself against, to stop it overwhelming him; echoes of Winnicott's false self. Young people who have been adopted might experience feelings of depression and a sense of emptiness and like Andrew, this might become particularly acute with the onset of adolescence. A study by Silverstein and Kaplan (1988), albeit rather dated but still relevant, identified seven core psychological/emotional issues for the adopted family, namely loss, rejection, shame, guilt, identity, intimacy and control. They go on to say that 'many adoptees as teens state that they truly have never felt close to anyone. Some declare a lifetime of emptiness related to a longing for the birth mother they may have never seen' (1982: 6).

Chess is a game of strategy, of attack and defence. It is a game of armies, but also families, the battleground overseen by the regal presence of the parental king and queen. Like families, the dynamics shift and change, the meaning and context of each piece in relation to another shifting as the game progresses. From a therapeutic perspective, it is a projective object sculpt of sorts – a family drama writ large – and playing chess with Andrew, I felt acutely aware of a parallel symbolic process, as he struggled to hold the line of defence against his intrusive thoughts and feelings. Andrew opened with the Queen's Gambit, a classic move that offers the sacrifice of the queen's pawn with the goal of gaining control of the centre ground. I was struck by the symbolism, of Andrew's own experience of being given up, and later I made the connection to myself with the television drama, the *Queen's Gambit*, which was the moving story of a child's experience of adoption, told through the medium of chess. I became very conscious of the act of 'taking' a pawn, the foot soldier 'child' of the chess family, removing it and placing it amongst the small, forlorn group of other taken pieces by the side of the board. Removed and placed elsewhere, like the adopted child (I have sometimes heard children describe adoption as being 'taken'). Likewise, the loss of the queen is momentous, a critical point, and moving into the end-game, Andrew would race his pawns across the board in a desperate attempt to regain his queen; to get mother back. Is that not the fantasy of all adopted children? At one stage, Andrew had two queens on the board, and I made a comment about there now being two mothers. And as we played, we spoke a little about his fear of death and dying – the ultimate check-mate – as the king is gradually rendered impotent by the opposing forces, cornered and powerless until the final, poignant act of submission – toppled – a small act of death.

As we played, I would make tentative observations, things I might notice about our game, about moves, his strategy, pieces being taken or protected, moves that signalled attack or defence or indeed withdrawal to a place of safety. An interesting paper by the psychotherapist Seitler (2016) talks about his experience of playing chess with a very non-verbal child, that ultimately facilitated an important process of disclosure. Like myself at times, Seitler questioned the value of the activity and his initial feelings of helplessness and disconnection and ultimately, whether what he was doing was good enough. Taking this to a clinical consultation, Seitler realised that the chess playing was indeed the therapy, that there was a process taking place, a conversation without words. Seitler talks about the notion of 'working obliquely' with troubled children, of the use of humour, banter and tentative commentary and how this 'allowed the child a way to find a play space s/he can claim as a thinking, imagining and speaking individual' (2016: 368). He goes on to say, 'often, my chitchat was met with little more than a grunt or two of acknowledgement. Nonetheless, it was acknowledgement all the same, on (the child's) part, of the existence of an outside world' (2016: 368).

Playing chess with Andrew during this 'in and out' conversation felt both poignant and deeply symbolic. On some level, albeit unconscious and unspoken, my profound sense was that we had found a safe way, a safe space, for him to communicate something of his experience. The very language of chess; of being moved, taken, swapped, replaced, attacked, defended, withdrawn, of mothers and fathers and death and resurrection, felt also to be the language of Andrew's adoptive experience.

Later in the session, Andrew chose to use the sandtray, the first time after many weeks that he had ever initiated a process of more spontaneous sensory/projective play. He filled small containers with water and sand, the contents frequently spilling out and overflowing. Amongst the box of various characters and objects by the sandtray, he found a figure of Harry Potter, and then a muscular wrestling figure, placing them in the sand facing each other, as if in combat – magic versus force. He found a small model of the Hulk and buried it in the sand and then poured water over it. Slowly excavating the Hulk, he was surprised and pleased to find a thick layer of wet sand sticking to the figure – 'look, he's got armour', he said. I commented on this, reflecting upon the Hulk's need for extra protection, given his already extreme strength. The Hulk is an interesting character in play therapy; the Freudian id of the Marvel Universe, the Hulk epitomises the primitive unconscious – a visceral brew of instinctive infantile rage, fight/flight and thalamic fear. By contrast, the Hulk's alter-ego, Dr Bruce Banner, is a man of logic and reason, a scientist with a highly developed cerebral cortex, all cognition and rational thought. Within a context of developmental trauma, the Hulk is a potent symbol. Amongst the box of various objects and figures, Andrew found a small baby's highchair and tried several times to push the Hulk figure down into the chair. He would not fit, and Andrew became frustrated, and the Hulk roared with rage, before being buried once again in the sand. Watching, I made a comment about the angry baby that was not getting what it needed. It was a fleeting moment of play, over in seconds, but somehow felt deeply significant; that Andrew had briefly let down his defensive shield and shown me something very important about his early experience. After the session, I wondered about the possible connections between the chess game and Andrew's sandplay; did one somehow facilitate the other?

Slight or moderate, occasionally rough, visibility good

Beyond Winnicott, the principle of 'good enough' (POGE) has spread across popular culture and beyond, becoming part of the vocabulary of everyday life; a conceptual antidote to the pursuit of perfection. Indeed, as Winnicott would argue, good enough is far better than perfection. I recently saw someone wearing a t-shirt that simply said 'good enough'. It is a phrase, dare I say a meme even, that people seem to intuitively understand and relate to, whether or not they are aware of its psychoanalytic origins. Interestingly, the good enough principle has also for some time now been a doctrine for software design, favouring agile, pragmatic, flexible and user-friendly design strategies that have long become a core part of our online support systems, an approach that eschews complexity and over-engineering. In many ways then, the notion of 'good enough' is something that has filtered and permeated into our everyday, collective cultural consciousness.

But good enough does not always feel good enough. I remember days after starting work as a university lecturer, chatting in the canteen to a senior academic colleague. He asked me about my undergraduate degree and which university I had gone to. It was a reasonable enough question, but meant that I had to explain that

I had not gone to university and did not have a degree. I glimpsed a brief, puzzled expression on my colleague's face as he grappled with this unexpected information and as I continued to dig a bigger hole in my self-esteem by telling him about dropping out of school, my years in the emotional wilderness and wayward life as a musician, I could see him glancing at his watch before announcing that he had an impending lecture to prepare for. I had outed myself and despite having a master's degree and having previously trained in social work and dramatherapy, I did not feel a member of the club. In truth, I had probably misinterpreted his hasty retreat, viewing it through my own, very particular, imposter-shaped lens.

I am not sure I feel comfortable with the term 'imposter syndrome'. Is it a syndrome? It is certainly neither a disease nor a disorder but more a colloquial term often used quite casually and with some abandon, sometimes made light of, sometimes downplayed, but also something that many people seem to be able to relate to at given times, particularly in the rather hierarchical structure of higher education. It is often given pejorative value, perceived negatively, although there might be some positive benefits or value to the imposter experience, perhaps in the form of internal drive or motivation. The actual term 'imposter syndrome' was first coined by Clance and Imes (1978) and can generally be defined as a psychological phenomenon characterised by intense feelings of intellectual fraudulence, a sense of unworthiness, that success has been simply down to luck and that one day your lack of skill and ability will be exposed – that you will be found out. As Sakulku (2011) states, pressures of perfectionism, increasing social comparisons and a fear of failure are all suggested as factors contributing to imposter syndrome and clearly there are connections here with feelings of not being good enough, although it is important to note that people experiencing imposter feelings do not generally hold a wider, negative self view. In this sense, the imposter phenomenon seems to exist within a specific professional context and role, or perhaps in relation to the perception of a particular set of skills and abilities.

But the imposter phenomenon is something I have often struggled with; feelings of being found out, that in some way I am not worthy of my professional role, that I have not earned it or, most of all, do not deserve it. It takes very little to tip me over into this position, a harmless question from a friendly colleague in the canteen is enough. It is a feeling that can sometimes paralyse me and sometimes (although not often) motivate me. The curious thing about the imposter phenomenon, from my experience, is that it can persist despite all evidence suggesting otherwise. Through a constant process of negative self-evaluation and self-imposed internal bias, I will dismiss praise and misattribute aspects of my own success to reinforce the sense that any achievements are unworthy and undeserved. There are links here with children who get referred for therapy and their own fears or expectations of failure – the not good enough child – who struggle with their motivation to do well and succeed. Perhaps adopted children like Andrew experience their own, particular version of imposter syndrome; a sense of not belonging. I have often wondered as to the extent that my own imposter feelings are linked to my early life experiences, my father's legacy, or something different and linked specifically to my academic role. Langford and Clance argue the case for early childhood, suggesting that 'people who experience impostor feelings are likely to come from families in which support for the individual is lacking, communications and behaviours are controlled by rules, and considerable conflict is present' (1993: 497). Or as Clance states – 'to truly understand the imposter phenomenon it is essential to start at the beginning – with the impostor's family' (1985: 465). But others (Gadsby, 2022) argue that the imposter phenomenon is more motivational than maladaptive, and that there might well be overlooked benefits to the phenomenon i.e. that an (albeit self-deceptive) belief in low ability creates a degree of motivational benefit that is 'particularly attractive for those who wish to succeed in contexts where the pathway to success is both challenging and opaque' (2022: 253).

Personally, whilst my own experience of imposter phenomenon has at times been a challenge to my professional identity and caused me considerable anxiety and self-doubt, it has in a sense always given me something to strive towards, or a current to swim against, which perhaps has not always been a bad thing. I have often had a very ambivalent relationship with academia, and it has not always felt to be a place where I easily fit or belong. I seem to be drawn to it and reject it in equal parts and in the end, I am content to feel something of an outsider – to not be a member of the club. As Olberding said, 'I sometimes still feel a fraud in academic environments, but neither do I mind it much' (2018).

I began this chapter talking about my early relationship with my father, the complex feelings of ambiguity around feeling loved or liked and the impact this has had on my sense of not being good enough. Yes, aspects of my childhood were certainly challenging; like the imposter, I have to an extent always felt an outsider, not quite sure where I fitted or belonged and like the advice that Winnicott gave my own father, I have to an extent also had to be my own father in the absence of a loving paternal relationship of my own. But in becoming a father myself I have also learned that it is possible to break these often very powerful generational patterns of being, that the past is not destined to be replayed and that scripts can be rewritten. But ultimately, my childhood is who I am and I would not have it any other way. My early, formative experiences have in a sense provided me with the drive and direction that have led to where I am today and for that, I am thankful. I am content to be good enough and also accepting that there are times when I am not good enough. This is, I guess, a part of the human condition. It is also what connects us to the children and families that we work with; that in the end, we are the same.

As some of you will have gathered, the rather cryptic headings for this chapter are taken from the 'Shipping Forecast', the BBC maritime broadcast, transmitted in the early hours, that provides reassuringly distinctive weather reports and forecasts for the seas around the coast of the British Isles. As an occasional insomniac, the 'Shipping Forecast' has been a comforting presence throughout my life; calm, dependable and mysteriously soothing. Through the pandemic, the growing climate emergency, illness and ongoing global political and financial turmoil, the shipping forecast remains a constant, unconditional companion, reaching out into the night and letting me know that the world is, indeed, good enough.

Recently, walking with my family on a beach in Cornwall, we watched a man row his dingy in from his tiny sailing yacht, moored a little way out from the beach. He methodically deflated his dingy, stowed it into his backpack and, our paths crossing, we got talking with him. He told us he was sailing around Britain, alone, having only learned to sail last year, with no support and for no reason beyond it was something he felt he needed to do. He was visibly shaking and explained that he had the 'jitters' – that he experienced acute bouts of anxiety at which point he had to come in, eat something, rest for a couple of days and try and build up his courage to continue. When we met him, he had been sailing for over two months and was just days away from his finish in North Devon. He was anxious that he would not make it, that the nearer he got to finishing the more likely it was that something would go wrong. We chatted to him for some time, took some photos for him and then bade each other farewell. I don't know if he ever made it, but feel sure he did. I often think of him, alone in his boat, isolated but not insulated, listening to the Shipping Forecast as it guided him safely around Britain's coastal waters. We have probably both been listening to the forecast at the same time. This was a man who did not think he was good enough to complete his magnificent adventure, but was on the home straight, battling his anxiety and doing something amazing. Good for him.

References

Abramovitch, H. (2021). When is it time to stop? When good enough becomes bad enough. *Journal of Analytical Psychology*, *66*(4), 907–925.

Clance, P. R. (1985). *The impostor phenomenon: Overcoming the fear that haunts your success*. Atlanta, GA: Peachtree (kindle version).

Clance, P. R., & Imes, S. A. (1978). The imposter phenomenon in high achieving women: Dynamics and therapeutic intervention. *Psychotherapy: Theory, Research & Practice*, *15*(3), 241–247.

Cozolino, L. (2004). *The making of a therapist: A practical guide for the inner journey*. New York: W. W. Norton & Company.

Gadsby, S. (2022). Imposter syndrome and self-deception. *Australasian Journal of Philosophy*, *100*(2), 247–261.

Langford, J., & Clance, P. R. (1993). The imposter phenomenon: Recent research findings regarding dynamics, personality and family patterns and their implications for treatment. *Psychotherapy: Theory, Research, Practice, Training*, *30*(3), 495–501.

Le Vay, A. D. (1970). Unpublished autobiography.

Le Vay, D. (2022). *Personal process in child-centred play therapy*. London: Routledge.

Olberding, A. (2018). *The Outsider*. Aeon URL = https://aeon.co/essays/how-useful-is-impostorsyndrome-in-academia.

Pitt, A. J. (2000). Hide and seek: The play of the personal in education. *Changing English*, *7*(1), 65–74.

Sachs, B. (2020). *On the importance of treatment failure*. www.pesi.co.uk/blog/2020/january/on-the-importance-of-treatment-failure (accessed on 7th November 2022).

Sakulku, J. (2011). The impostor phenomenon. *International Journal of Behavioral Science*, *6*(1), 75–97.

Seitler, B. N. (2016). When words were wanted, but woefully wanting, we waged war with chess. *The American Journal of Psychoanalysis*, *76*, 362–375.

Silverstein, D. N., & Kaplan, S. (1988). *Lifelong issues in adoption*. In Coleman, K. T. L., Hornby H., & Boggis, C. (Eds.), *Working with older adoptees: A source book of innovative models* (pp. 45–53). Portland. University of Southern Maine.

Winnicott, D. W. (1953). Transitional objects and transitional phenomena – A study of the first not-me possession. *International Journal of Psycho-Analysis*, *34*, 89–97.

Winnicott, D. W. (1965). *Communicating and not communicating leading to a study of certain opposites*. The Maturational Processes and the Facilitating Environment: Studies in the Theory of Emotional Development. Madison, CT: International Universities.

Wright, F. (2022). Shame: Healing and beyond. In D. Le Vay & E. Cuschieri (Eds.), *Personal process in child-centred play therapy* (pp. 74–90). London: Routledge.

Postcards from the playroom

There was a time when I was employed in a dual role, as a social worker and a therapist. The two roles were not necessarily that compatible and it was not always easy to protect and maintain the boundaries around my therapist role. I was working in a Family Centre, a fantastic place that provided early, preventative, therapeutic and social care support to children and families. Twice a week we would provide lunch for parents and their young, pre-school children. We would all sit and eat together, like a large extended family, supporting the adults in their parenting skills and proving important play opportunities for the children. In their wisdom, the local authority decided to close all the Family Centres across the county, one of the biggest and most damaging acts of policy short-sightedness that I have seen, the legacy of which continues many years later.

We often undertook home visits and I recall once visiting the family of a boy that I was also working with therapeutically. It was a very deprived family, materially and emotionally, the consequence of acute generational neglect. The boy answered the door and wordlessly handed me a picture that he had drawn. I invited him to tell me about the picture and he explained that it was the two of us, him and me, being carried away in a hot air balloon, far away into the sky. I still have the picture and I often think of this boy and our fantastic adventures of his imagination.

Chapter 5

I walk, therefore I am

Paths to self-care

I taught for many years on an MA Play Therapy programme. It was a two-year programme and towards the end of the students training, I always included a 'lecture' that began, somewhat randomly, with me sharing photographs of my various long-distance hiking adventures. It is fair to say that I had what might be best described as a rather idiosyncratic approach to teaching; anything to avoid the more standardised lecture format, which my ever-present imposter voice told me I was not very good at anyway. Some of the students looked puzzled, some curious, some intrigued and some no doubt just a little alarmed. Where on earth was this going? Why isn't he telling me how to deal with that child on placement who every week wants to squeeze paint on my head and urinate in the sandtray? Why won't he just tell us what to do?

But regardless, I would press on with my little slide show, sharing with the students my story of hiking 866 kilometres along the entire length of the French Pyrenees, on the GR10 trail that runs west to east from the Atlantic to the Mediterranean. It was a journey that took two months to complete and was no doubt one of the most challenging, risky, gruelling, joyful, demanding, tedious and emotionally exhilarating experiences of my life. I shared photographs of the Tour du Mont Blanc, hiking around the largest mountain in Europe and of scrabbling and scrambling across the rugged mountain interior of Corsica on the infamous GR20, the toughest long-distance hike in Europe. And then there was trekking across Mallorca, running around Menorca and hiking the Atlantic coast of Portugal, along the Fisherman's Trail, in the delightful company of my daughter.

I talked to the students about mountain paths so narrow and vertiginous that it felt like I might fall to my doom at any moment; having to find a good enough handhold on the perilous GR20 to prevent me sliding 30 feet down the mountainside. I talked about getting lost and finding my way. I talked about the importance of detailed maps in getting a sense of the relief of the land; the shape, contours and configuration of the landscape that we were walking in – the high points and low points. I talked about how the sight of a stone cairn at 3000 metres in driving rain and practically zero visibility might be the difference between life and death. I talked about the exhilaration of taking risks, of ignoring the guide books and taking a different route. I talked about finding one's limits and knowing one's boundaries.

DOI: 10.4324/9781003352563-5

I talked about the importance of having the right resources; the boots, clothes, medical kit and my deep attachment to my trusty hiking stick. I talked about the deep, exhausted satisfaction of completing a challenging day on the trail and of the relentless tedium of repetition and of having to walk through the pain of failing knees and blistered feet. I talked about wanting to give up and how hard it was at times to carry on, of missing my family and how on occasion it was only the relationship and support of my fellow hikers that gave me the strength to continue. And of course, as I continued with my rather quirky slideshow of a lecture, the students soon realised that I was indeed talking to them about the child that wants to squeeze paint over their heads and urinate in the sandtray. Metaphor is a wonderful thing.

Paths to recovery and self-care

Before I set out on my two-month trek along the Pyrenees, people often asked me why I was doing it. The obvious answer was, well . . . why not? As many mountain climbers might say, because it was there. In truth, there was something of a mid-life crisis moment about it. I was in my mid-40s at the time, in fact my mid-everything; middle-aged, middle-sized, middle-class, middle-income, and I felt I needed to do something to haul myself out of the middle-sized, existential shaped black hole that I was slowly but surely disappearing into. I did no preparation, no training and the longest distance I had previously walked was a fifteen-mile school sponsored walk with my mother, when I was about 12 years old. As many people pointed out before I set off, it was either very brave or very stupid. To be fair, most said stupid.

But there was also something else. I was working at the time as a play therapist for a specialist local authority organisation providing treatment and assessment for children and young people with sexually harmful behaviour. The team manager had left a year previously and not been replaced and as the only full-time member of the team I found myself in the position of acting manager and, on reflection, I think I was pretty burnt out. It was challenging, stressful, anxious and disturbing work, at the very heart of which lay the need to manage and tolerate very high levels of risk. Perhaps I was running away, or at least walking away, a sort of slow-motion version of fight and flight. So, I negotiated a three-month unpaid break and, with the blessing of my family, disappeared for two months into the heat and mist of the Pyrenean mountains.

There is a certain stealth about vicarious trauma, it creeps up on you, silently, unbeknown. It is there before you realise it. I am not sure as to the extent that this was my experience, but there is clearly a cost to empathic connection with traumatised children. To empathise with another's suffering, to validate their experience and to feel it as if it were your own creates a vulnerability in us as clinicians – indeed it is this very vulnerability and capacity to connect that lies at the heart of being an effective therapist. As Clark (1980) says, empathy can be defined as that 'unique capacity of the human being to feel the experiences, needs, aspirations, frustrations, sorrows, joys, anxieties, hurt or hunger as if they were his or her own' (1980: 190). As play therapists, working with children who have experienced severe trauma and abuse, there is a need to step repeatedly into their worlds, to find a point of connection. More than just listening to children's stories, this demands that we inhabit and live their stories, through role play, dramatic enactment and projective/sensory play. These are often messy, sticky, confused, chaotic and visceral worlds of victims and monsters, flooded sandtrays, deadly potions, characters held powerless and immobile. As well as young children with sexually problematic behaviours, I also worked with adolescent and adult sexual offenders and looking back, with the benefit of distance and perspective, I can understand more now about the impact this work had on me, although it was not so obvious at the time. It is a little like going for a walk late in the day, as the light begins to fade. It is only when you get home and look out of the window that you realise just how dark it really was outside.

I had difficulty sleeping (still do, in fact), had bad dreams, was often anxious and experienced intrusive thoughts and feelings. I over-worried about the safety and well-being of my own young daughter, needing to know that her violin teacher, gymnastics teacher, or whichever teacher it might be, had been appropriately vetted and police checked. I developed a rather distorted and overly bleak world view in which everyone was a potential perpetrator. In my darkest, most disturbing dreams even I was an abuser, the trauma of the work seeping into my unconscious. Always being somewhat prone to pessimism, this easily spilled over into cynicism; a deep mistrust of the world around me and while naturally (and happily) introverted by nature, I was susceptible to becoming emotionally isolated and disconnected. It is something of a paradox that a professional role that requires such a deep level of emotional connection can leave one feeling so disconnected. Of course, I could understand this rationally within an analytic frame of projective identification and countertransference; that my feelings of anxiety, disconnection and existential nihilism were a powerful communication of the child's internal world, but I was affected by it nonetheless – knowing is sometimes not enough.

Consciously and unconsciously, formally and informally, I found ways to moderate and mitigate the impact of the work. Clinical supervision and personal therapy were, of course, important, but other places and spaces held equal importance. Our family allotment became a wonderful place for cathartic processing; digging, weeding and growing. Research (Lowry et al., 1987) has suggested that digging around in the dirt is an effective antidepressant, the 'friendly' microbes in the soil activating the production of serotonin. So yes, gardening really does make us happy. I spent a wonderful few weeks building a shed in the woods backing onto our allotment out of old wooden pallets and various other bits of recycled material. The rather mindless process of creating something from nothing was a joy and I often reflect upon this time with deep, nostalgic affection. Sublimation is a wonderful defence mechanism. And the symbolism of building a shelter in the woods does not escape me; it is clearly what I needed and took me back to building dens as a young child – a safe place to hide away. The allotment was a place where I could happily, if you will forgive the pun, lose the plot, and disengage from the rather invasive nature of my clients' storied lives.

Running was also an important form of emotional and physical release, especially relevant within the context of working with childhood trauma. Children who have experienced relational trauma are unable to either fight or run, their brains flooded with cortisol and norepinephrine. The helplessness of the traumatised child is often felt by the therapist, a form of counter-dissociation one could say and the experience of being able to run, to discharge the build-up of stress, can be helpful. Back in the day, when I was still able to run long distances, I cherished the experience of being able to lose myself in my running, to insulate myself from the outside world. There is something of a dissociative quality about running. Responding to questions about what he thought about as he ran, the writer (and marathon runner) Haruki Murakami said, 'I always ponder the question. What exactly do I think about when I am running? I don't have a clue' (2009: 16). I think there is a lot to be said for not having a clue.

But both despite (and because of) my initial and rather extreme Pyrenean initiation it is walking, particularly long-distance hiking, that has really become an integral part of my life. I walk therefore I think; I think therefore I am. Therefore, I walk and . . . I am. This, in shorthand, is my philosophy about hiking; that in a strange sense I walk myself into existence. Robert Macfarlane, in his wonderful book *The Old Ways*, talked about his sense of 'walking as enabling sight and thought rather than encouraging retreat and escape; paths that offer not only means of traversing space, but also ways of feeling, being and knowing' (2013: 24). The well-worn mountain paths that I, and so many others have followed, have literally been walked into the ground over many hundreds of years; they connect us together in body and mind, to the past, present and future. The path leads us around, but also back. It takes us both outside and inside. We are all time travellers, metaphysically, as we move back and forth along a continuum of past experiences and possible futures, just as walking leads one to all sorts of junctures, crossroads, encounters, signposts and route-markers. Paths, as Macfarlane says, run through people as surely as they run through places – 'walking is not the action by which one arrives at knowledge; it is itself the means of knowing' (2013:17).

The four-pebble problem

Walking has long been linked to creativity. The philosopher Nietzsche wrote that, 'all truly great thoughts are conceived by walking' (1889: 34) and one can walk Nietzsche's Path, the winding trail that connects the medieval mountain village of Eze with the coast of the French Cote D'Azur. Charles Darwin famously engaged in daily walks along the gravel 'sandwalk' at Down House, his home in Kent, as he contemplated his theory of natural selection. He referred to it as his 'thinking path' and the story goes that Darwin always ensured that he had a small pile of pebbles on the path, thoughtfully kicking one with each turn around the circuit. Some of the more complex ideas he grappled with were known as 'four-pebble problems'. I think we have all grappled with our respective four-pebble problems.

The philosopher Rousseau wrote that 'I am unable to reflect when I am not walking: the moment I stop, I think no more and as soon as I am again in motion, my head resumes its working' (1891:72). And the poet Wallace Stevens wrote, with a sense of poignant precision, that 'perhaps, the truth depends on a walk around a lake' (Locke, 1993: 195). My personal motto is, if in doubt, go for a walk, and I know that at times when I feel stuck, blocked or uninspired it is invariably the act of walking that frees something up, that loosens my thinking and enables me to capture something that has previously felt infuriatingly elusive. My premise then, is that cognition is motion sensitive, or to put it a little more cryptically, walking enables us to think about not thinking.

The neuroscientist Arne Dietrich (2006) coined the rather wonderful term 'transient hypofrontality' that describes how during physical activity, such as walking or running (or even, I might suggest, digging at the allotment), the brain's neural resources are 'down-regulated' in order to direct bodily motion. The activity of the prefrontal cortex is minimised, so allowing a process of spontaneous creativity. Dietrich suggests that this slowdown of the deliberate attention system allows unconscious thoughts of a more random, unfiltered, unusual or even bizarre nature to surface and become more represented within working memory. The part of the brain's function that would normally judge or censor the appropriateness of certain thoughts and ideas is potentially less active, so allowing for more novel, unconventional, unorthodox and left-field ideas to emerge. This links to interesting research (Oppezzo & Schwartz, 2014) that suggests that walking boosts creative ideation by up to 60%. A particularly striking aspect of this research was that the environment was not a key factor; the dramatic increase in creative ideation was the same whether someone was walking outside in the open countryside or on a treadmill in a gymnasium.

Whilst walking on a treadmill might be very beneficial, there is also something uniquely both mindful and mindless about walking in nature. It slows us down, allows for the act of noticing: the translucent morning dew on a spider's web; the ephemeral shimmer of a mayfly's silvery wing; the veins of a yellowing, autumn leaf; the distant, high-pitched keen of a red kite; the pungent, earthy smell of oakmoss. The act of noticing is important and, of course, it is what we do all the time as play therapists. I am writing this having just returned from a session with a 9-year-old boy. He was tired and it was a particularly quiet session and sometimes when I am not sure what else to say I simply notice things out loud. I noticed his new haircut, his yawn, his slight reticence about going to the playroom, his tentative step due to a sore foot, the drawing on the back of his hand. There is a lot to be said for simply noticing. To notice is to be present, to be present is to be attuned, and to be attuned is to be connected.

An extensive scoping review (Mau et al., 2021) of studies examining the potential psychological benefits of long-distance walking in adults concluded that there were clear links to positive mental health and particularly in the alleviation of emotional distress. From a personal perspective, this resonates with my own experience of walking as being an important part of my self-care process. As a counterpoint to the previously mentioned Oppezzo and Schwartz study, this review also concluded that the combination of the health benefits of physical activity and time spent in nature were indicators of the therapeutic value of walking, and neuroimaging studies indicated that walking through natural environments (as compared to walking in urban environments) may lead to reduced neural activity in an area of the brain associated with mental illness. Similarly, the review pointed towards a growing body of literature revealing the harmonising impact of nature exposure on physiological stress reactions. So, perhaps the truth does depend upon a walk around a lake.

Walking in natural environments is an experience of sensory immersion and as said, this allows one to become more present with the world around us. But walking is also an embodied experience, enabling a deep connection with one's own physicality. The body communicates its aches and pains, its points of strength and vulnerability. When I have been on long distance hikes over a period of days or weeks, I have experienced a deep sense of internal, physical attunement; the beginnings of a blister, the ache of a knee joint, the insistent beat of a raised heart level, the sensation of the ground beneath my feet. At times there is a flow about walking, a sense of fluidity and ease in which mind, body, spirit and the external world feel completely in tune. At other times, I feel disconnected, uncoordinated, my legs heavy and cumbersome, my gait awkward. As existential psychologist Rollo May suggests, 'it is amazing how many hints and guides and intuitions for living come to the sensitive person who has ears to hear what (their) body is saying' (1953: 76).

Interestingly, May wrote extensively about courage, not in the sense of the warrior who must disregard or supress their anxiety, fears and doubts in order to march into battle, but more about small acts of internal courage, the confrontation of those things that might influence our internal psychological make-up and unconscious patterns of relating – 'the inhibitions, repressions and childhood conditionings' (1953: 119) that govern our feelings, thoughts and behaviours. Rather than ignoring fear, May saw courage as the active exploration of fear, including the sense of listening to, and with, one's body. This is perhaps analogous to aspects of long-distance walking; the opening up to one's internal process, the allowing of unconscious thoughts and feelings to spontaneously arise, the act of having to confront and engage with one's fears and anxieties as they might emerge and the letting go of the familiar routines and structures that might otherwise govern and structure our lives. To be in one's own company for long periods of time is not always easy and might well demand the embracing (and tolerance) of uncertainty. And connecting and being sensitive to what our bodies are communicating to us might also be an act of courage. On a long-distance hike, the mind and body are in a constant conversation, sometimes perhaps more of an argument, although the experience of pain and exertion is not necessarily negative and indeed 'may have meaning by being incorporated into notions of self-reliance and self-care' (Mau et al., 2023: 7).

This does, I believe have relevance for us as therapists, the being of which also takes courage, and in many ways, we are talking here about the personhood of the therapist and the development of self-awareness, insight and reflexivity, or what May (1953) termed 'meta-perspective' – the ability to view ourselves from a distance, or from multiple perspectives and positions. This links, I think, with aspects of Rogers' (1951) model of person-centred therapy and Maslow's (1962) concept of self-actualisation. Beyond self-care, important enough in itself, the therapeutic benefits of walking are also then bound up in the process of becoming a person and the sense, as said earlier, of walking oneself into existence. This in turn, I would suggest, connects with our capacity to be resilient, robust and self-aware person-centred therapists. Furthermore, the experience of becoming 'body-aware' and attuned to one's physicality is intrinsic to the embodied process of psychotherapy, of particular importance I would suggest to play therapists working within the realm of the non-verbal. Play therapy, as in psychotherapy more generally, takes place within the intersubjective space between therapist and child. If we accept Crossley's assertion that the body is the 'very basis of human subjectivity' (1995: 44) then we need to be attuned to the embodied communication that is such an integral part of the therapeutic process.

The notion of the body being the very basis of human subjectivity might well hold very particular significance for some people. A study by Calsius et al. (2019) explored the long-distance walking experience of people with multiple sclerosis and found that the physical effort significantly enhanced their perceptions of what their bodies were capable of. Rather than being governed by the limitations of their bodies, participants felt that their bodies became a source of 'strength, joy, and meaningfulness', and that the pushing of their physical limits was empowering. Similar findings (Lesser et al., 2020) emerged from research with cancer survivors, where the 'physical effort of long-distance walking served as a reminder for some of how they were in fact strong, as opposed to what the disease may have implied to them' (Lesser et al., 2020). What underlines or underpins these findings seems to be that 'bodily accomplishment is intimately tied to mental states or notions of self' (Mau et al., 2022: 7).

This has a specific resonance with my personal experience of having been recently diagnosed with Parkinson's Disease. I am acutely aware at times of the very profound disconnect between mind and body – a very awkward, disjointed conversation – and my sense of having to 'push through' a protesting, resistant body before reaching a point of ease and comfort. But at other times I experience a sense of freedom and the liberating experience of not feeling physically defined by my condition. Also, my attitude to the purpose and value of walking has shifted since my diagnosis. Physical exercise is a critical part of the management of Parkinson's and so now walking has taken on new meaning; it is in itself a form of treatment and self-medication. But Parkinson's aside, there have also been times when I have relished the experience (and pain) of putting my body through some quite extreme physical challenges, almost like some kind of masochistic release. Although not religious, I could perhaps describe my experiences of long-distance hiking as a form of secular pilgrimage and whilst these journeys are imbued with a great sense of satisfaction, accomplishment, meaning and discovery, there is invariably also a degree of suffering and pain, which on reflection I am rather curious about.

Egan (2011) used the term 'the body as a memorial' to suggest that the physical strain and discomfort that long-distance walkers expose themselves to could be an expression, conscious or otherwise, of the personal struggles they may be going through. In this sense, the 'wounded soul of the walker may attain a more concrete form in the wounded body and the pain associated with long-distance walking may be a vicarious expression of the pain one might be feeling psychologically' (Mau et al., 2022: 7). Much has been written about the relationship between the body and trauma (Ogden et al., 2006; van der Kolk, 2015) and this takes us back to the notion of vicarious trauma and the physical, psychological and emotional responses to working with highly traumatised children. As I have said, there is a personal legacy of this work, for both better and worse. We carry it with us: the children in our pocket and the burdened rucksack on our back.

In good company

Walking for me can be both a solitary and shared experience, but for long-distance hiking over a period of days and even weeks, I have always sought the companionship of fellow hikers, friends with whom I can share the experience. Whilst by nature I am prone to introversion, which one might think of as a good quality for the solitary walker, this can easily tip into a rather more brooding process of introspection and even melancholia that can all too easily leave me feeling disconnected, detached and disenchanted. When I was younger, in my early 20s, I recall going on a solo walking trip to the Lake District with the expressed intention (as I explained to my partner) of 'finding myself', whatever I thought that might mean. In truth, I did not like too much what I found and returned after a few days with my existential tail between my aching legs, feeling rather sorry for myself. It is something of a paradox, but as an introvert, I rather like being around people. It is a fallacy that introverts do not like other people's company and eschew social contact, in fact this is very important, but personally I tend to prefer the social intimacy of one-to-one relationships or small groups, or to be able to dip in and out of larger social situations. Interestingly, I think this is partly why my training took me from dramatherapy to play therapy, preferring the intimacy of individual work to the more outward-facing demands of groupwork. And of course, rather than either/ or, the dynamics of introversion and extroversion are understood much more now (like so many other aspects of our neurodiverse world) as being context-dependent and existing more as a spectrum rather than a polarised continuum.

As well as the physical demands required, long-distance hiking over a period of days, weeks and even months is a test of one's emotional and psychological resilience – a test that I have not always passed with flying colours. Walking in the Pyrenees for two months, there were many times when I felt like giving up, whether due to pain, tedium, exhaustion or most of all missing my family. At these times, my good friend and walking companion would talk to me, support me, give me encouragement or simply just listen to me complaining. At other times, I would do the same for him, when he felt he had had enough and felt like giving up. It was our relationship that got us through and neither of us, I guess, would have been able to complete the journey on our own. It was a test of our friendship; we laughed, cried, joked, argued, but most of all, survived – celebrating the highs and hauling each other through the lows. We met many people along the way; good people that we walked with often for days and weeks and many of them gave up at some stage, due to physical or emotional reasons. Sometimes my friend and I walked together, chatting amiably and sometimes we walked in an easy silence. Sometimes we walked with a little distance between us, an unsaid balancing act of mutual proximity that recognised and respected our unspoken desire for occasional silence and solitude. In essence, we negotiated a way of being together, mindful of our respective needs and wants. This is, of course, much like the relational process of therapy – sometimes feeling connected and sometimes distant, but over time establishing a relationship that feels contained, safe and trustworthy.

Some thoughts on survival

On the trail, my rucksack was both my friend and my enemy. It sustained me with food, warmth and shelter, but also weighed me down, pulled at my shoulders and dug into my back. It was both a help and a hindrance, so my attachment to this home upon my back was ambivalent, to say the least. Walking was a constant process of readjusting straps to ease tension and redistribute the weight. I would also do anything I could to lighten the load and anything that was deemed unnecessary was mercilessly jettisoned along the way; books, clothes, used maps, tin whistles, food sometimes and in one occasion of particular weakness, the bright orange survival bag that I was carrying. Midway through the trip, when high up on a very exposed mountain ridge section of the trail, we were in danger of being caught up by a violent thunder storm. Pursued by spectacular lightning strikes and mighty cracks of thunder, we ran the last few kilometres in a desperate attempt to get to the safety of the refuge before the storm overtook us. At one point, my friend stopped and said that if the storm caught up with us while we were so exposed, we might have to resort to finding a sheltered spot and using our survival bags to climb into and wait it out. 'Ah, well . . . about that', I muttered shamefully into the heaving wind, as I confessed that I had thrown it away some days ago to save space and weight in my rucksack. I will not repeat here what he called me, only to say that I deserved every word of it.

On the Tour du Mont Blanc, a 170-kilometre ten-day trek that circumnavigates the iconic mountain, we were forecast two weeks of hot, September sun. I decided I did not need my raincoat and waterproof trousers and left them behind, opting instead for my lightweight poncho, which had served me well in the past. For nine days the weather was sunny and hot. On the final day, the temperature dropped by around 20 degrees and high up at over 2000 metres on the trail it began to rain, sleet and snow. Under my poncho I was just wearing a t-shirt and shorts and before long I was drenched and freezing and was so cold that I lost all feeling in my hands and fingers. All I could do was to alternate between using one hand to hold my hiking stick and keeping the fingers of my other hand in my mouth, in a desperate attempt to stop them from freezing. It was not a great look. My two friends non-chalantly paused to put on their waterproofs. They were warm and dry and happy to take their time, but I could feel my body temperature plunging and decided to go on alone to get to the shelter and warmth of our accommodation as quickly as possible. In no time, I was enveloped by a deep veil of thick mist, with visibility down to just a few feet and I had no map or compass. Gentle mountain streams had in seconds turned into raging, precarious torrents. This is it, I thought. If I take one wrong turning, I could get lost, be swept away or die of hyperthermia, or possibly a combination of all three. It was an anxious moment and I decided, knowing that I was at that point standing on the right path, to simply stop and wait, in the freezing rain, until someone else came along, who I could tag along with and get to safety. It was probably only about fifteen minutes, although felt like hours, but eventually a well-equipped American couple came by and I walked with them for the last few miles to the welcome, dry warmth of a cable car station. In the station there were some public toilets, including a hand dryer and I stood for some time warming my hands and my spirit. To this day, years on, I cannot use a hand dryer without recalling this experience. I also lose the feeling in my fingers very quickly in cold weather, and often wonder if this is due to some kind of nerve damage from my Mont Blanc experience.

On the GR20, a highly challenging hike/scramble across the rugged mountains of central Corsica, there was one particular day that required a very demanding ascent up Mount Cinto, the highest point on the island. The weather was closing in and having been shaken by a rather dramatic fall the previous day, I and another of our group decided to take an alternative lower-level variant, taking us around rather than over the mountain. Having learned my lesson in the Pyrenees and also made a pledge to my family not to take unnecessary risks I decided, on this occasion, to take the safer option. Conversely, I recall a day in the Eastern Pyrenees when we were approaching Mount Canigou, an impressively imposing 2780m mountain. Whilst our guidebook clearly indicated taking a low level but longer route around the mountain, my walking companion (with a glint in his eye) said, 'what the hell, let's just go over the top'. And so, over the top we went, pausing at the summit for a restorative hot drink and magnificent views across the plains of Roussillon and our distant goal of the Mediterranean.

What I have learned from these experiences, the moral of the story perhaps, is that it is important to think about our safety needs; whether this be in terms of hiking or clinical practice. We need to practise self-care and learn to value ourselves and be attuned to the needs of both ourselves and our clients. We need the right resources to be able to work safely, be they physical, emotional or psychological. The loads we carry as therapists, like my rucksack, will weigh us down; burden us with feelings of clinical responsibility, risk, too little time and too big a case-load. We need to think carefully about our survival bags, even if this requires investment, attention and commitment. The oft repeated mantra of my friend in the Pyrenees, whilst rightly admonishing me for jettisoning important resources, was to 'never mess with the mountains' and perhaps the same can be said of therapy. Certainly, there are times as therapists when we feel enveloped by fog or caught in a storm, unable to see clearly, afraid of getting lost or being swept away by the raging currents. There are times to take risks and times to be cautious. Whichever, we have an ethical responsibility, both to our clients and ourselves, to ensure that we have the resources available to support and guide us through these moments.

Some thoughts on cairns

The stacking of one individual object on top of another object i.e. the stacking of bricks or the beginnings of tower construction is a key milestone in infant development, with 75% of infants being able to build a two-block tower at the age of 15 months. At the age of 18 months, 50% of infants are able to build a five-block tower (Marcinowski et al., 2016). This emergent skill of object construction is a particularly unique aspect of development, as the infant explores and experiments with the conceptual awareness of creating something new from different objects, each of which might have distinct properties and qualities from one another. It is the development of skills of visual, spatial and motor coordination. It is also the beginning of symbolic play wherein individual bricks, or indeed the tower itself, might be a representation of something else i.e. an object can have another symbolic meaning. There is something quite primal about the placing of one block on top of another, both in terms of infant development but also in terms of societal development; the beginnings of early structures that might have practical or symbolic significance.

This brings to mind the stone cairn, a structure as old as humanity itself. There is a beautiful simplicity about a cairn, these reassuringly weathered, enigmatic stacks of stone and rock that rise like abstract sculptures from the ground, both small and large. They are aesthetically pleasing, enduring, organic creations of various styles, shapes and sizes, reminding me of a craggy, oversized Jenga tower or object sculpt of sorts; an expression of gravity-defying projective play pushing up from the base of a sandtray, as if a giant, mythic child has been at play in the open wilds of the mountains. But of course, cairns also have an important purpose and function. On hiking trails, they serve as route markers, invariably sitting at junctions on the path, indicating to the passing walker the direction of travel. Many times, in rain or mist or the gathering folds of the fading mountain light, a cairn has been the difference between a right and a wrong turn, a choice that could have serious consequences.

As hikers pass by, some add a stone to the cairn, often in thoughtful contemplation; an expression of gratitude to those who have gone before and a communication to those yet to pass, an unspoken message from one hiker to the next. In this sense, the cairn becomes part of the narrative of the trail, conversation pieces, points of connection. They hold the living history of the route, connecting past, present and future. Hikers will often gather by a cairn; a time to pause and reflect, to share stories, to give advice, eat, consult maps and tend to blisters. They form a point of intersection, the crossing of paths, the telling of what has gone before and what is to come. Cairns also mark the highpoint of the day, a symbol of achievement and reassurance that the hard upward work has been done. Many times, after hours of aching ascent and demoralising false summits, that cruelest of mountain teases, it has been the sight of the cairn in the far distance that has given me the drive to continue, knowing that respite (and lunch) is near.

As well as the highpoint, cairns might also mark the crossing point, the transition between borders, from one country or region, to the next. These are often wild open spaces, exposed and exposing, the hiker a tiny figure against the sweeping grandeur of the mountain landscape. These are liminal spaces, the threshold between one space and another. They mark changes of language, currency, culture, geography but also perhaps points of internal change, shifts in perspective; the stark, dramatic relief of the mountains proving an external counterpoint to one's internal landscape. I have often felt moved by the vast, impressionistic nature of these places, all the more so for the effort it has taken to reach them.

Cairns can also be memorial sites and burial markers. Walking on the Tour du Mont Blanc, I passed a cairn marking the spot where a young hiker was struck and killed by lightning, a sombre reminder of the dangers that mountains can hold. Passing hikers would sometimes add a stone, a collective act of remembrance. The building of cairns goes back to the beginning of time, the stone mounds sometimes containing burial chambers and there is rich history of folklore, myth and legend, often connected with grief, loss and mourning. In Scottish Highland folklore, it was said that before battle, each man would place a stone in a pile. Those who survived the battle and returned home would remove a stone from the pile. The stones that remained, a symbol of the missing, were built into a cairn to honour the dead. In Portugal, a cairn is called a *moledro*. Legend has it that the moledros are enchanted soldiers, and if one stone is taken from the pile and put under a pillow, in the morning a soldier will appear for a brief moment, then will change back to a stone and magically return to the pile. According to Greek mythology, the god Hermes, messenger and protector of travellers, was put on trial by Hera for slaying the serpent monster, Argus. The rest of the gods, acting as jury, were given pebbles to throw at whoever they thought was in the right. Hermes, having argued his case so skilfully was buried under a pile of pebbles, so becoming the first cairn. Perhaps in this sense the cairn represents a symbol of truth.

The stone structures are ubiquitous throughout culture, with a rich diversity of legend and folklore reaching across Africa, the Middle East, Asia and the Americas. It is this universality and cultural breadth that gives the humble cairn, a simple pile of stones, such poignant, symbolic value and meaning. Perhaps the cairn can also hold a meaning for us as therapists; symbolic markers of our own particular pathways; points of transition, change, losses and gains; markers that prevent us from losing our way. Similarly, they might symbolise something about the therapeutic process, fixed reference points that can help both therapist and client navigate their way together through often challenging terrain of the therapeutic landscape. It is also interesting to see how frequently cairn-like structures appear in play therapy, often within the process of sandplay, towers of bricks, sand, wooden blocks, Lego; archetypal shapes and forms drawn deep from the collective unconscious. Recently, I had a session with a 10-year-old adopted child. He began the session by placing a tiny figure in the base of the sandtray, enclosed in a small wooden box, and then drawing up the wet sand in a large mound around the buried figure. On top of the mound, he created a tower of wooden bricks, a marker of sorts. My strong sense was that of a burial chamber and I was struck by the symbolism, wondering about the tiny figure that lay deep within this chamber. Just as many cairns in the natural world are markers of grief and loss, I wondered about the potential meaning of this child's poignant act of remembrance and who or what he might be grieving for. Himself perhaps.

On a final thought about cairns, it is important to note that there has been a recent trend towards artistic rock stacking and balancing, with people drawn to the aesthetic and, for some, spiritual significance of the stone structures. Whilst acknowledging the creative process at play and that there is indeed a delight in coming across these gravity defying structures, this is potentially problematic as they could confuse hikers for whom cairns can be an important navigational aid. For others, there are issues around the disruption of the local ecology and natural landscape of an area. So, my message would be to be aware and mindful of the context, meaning and purpose of the cairn, their role, value and cultural significance, the principal message for all hikers being that of 'leave no trace' and to not disturb the natural environment that they are walking through.

Final steps

My experience of long-distance walking is that it is always the day's last few miles that are the hardest, as one starts to anticipate the ending; a cold beer, hot shower, good food and an opportunity to rest aching legs and sore feet. Just as one thinks the end is in sight there is invariably one last hill to climb, a tedious road walk, a tricky scrambling descent or unexpected diversion. I think as therapists we can all relate to this. There is both exhaustion and satisfaction, pain and relief and short respite before beginning again. Endings are hard.

Ending this chapter has also been hard – sometimes it is about knowing when to stop. It has, in keeping with the theme, been something of a diversionary piece, a tangential foray, one might say, so thank you for staying with me. There is, I believe, a truth to be found in walking, whatever that might be, and I thank the students to whom I subjected my idiosyncratic lecture/slide show for indulging me. I hope also they got a sense of what I was talking about when I was talking about walking, to paraphrase Murakami (2009). The essence of this chapter has been about self-care. For me this has been walking, but for others it might be something very different; pottery, theatre, music, gardening perhaps. Find what works for you, and do it. Embrace your 'transient hypofrontality'.

References

Calsius, J. et al. (2019). Wandering through the desert with multiple sclerosis: How outdoor life recalibrates body awareness and self-identity. *Journal of Interdisciplinary and Multidisciplinary Research, 3*(1), 37–77.

Clark, K. B. (1980). Empathy: A neglected topic in psychological research. *American. Psychologist, 35*, 18.

Crossley, N. (1995). Merleau-Ponty, the elusive body and carnal society. *Body and Society, 1*, 43–63.

Dietrich, A. (2006). Transient hypofrontality as a mechanism for the psychological effects of exercise. *Psychiatry Research.* November 29, *145*(1), 79–83.

Egan, K. (2011). I want to feel the Camino in my legs: Trajectories of walking on the Camino de Santiago. In A. Fedele & R. L. Blanes (Eds.), *Encounters of body and soul in contemporary religious practices: Anthropological reflections* (pp. 3–22). New York and Oxford: Berghahn Books.

Lesser, I. A. et al. (2020). A mixed-methods evaluation of a group-based trail walking program to reduce anxiety in group of cancer survivors. *Applied Cancer Research, 40*(1), 1–10.

Locke, K. E. (Ed.) (1993). *Wallace Stevens: The art of impermanence.* Bloomington, IN: Indiana University Press.

Lowry. C. A., Hollis, J. et al. (1987). Identification of an immune-responsive mesolimbocortical serotonergic system: Potential role in regulation of emotional behavior. *Neuroscience, 146*(2), 756–772 (accessed on 11th May 11 2007).

Macfarlane, R. (2013). *The old ways: A journey on foot.* London: Penguin.

Marcinowski, E., Campbell, J., Faldowski, R., & Michel, G. F. (2016). Do hand preferences predict stacking skill during infancy? *Developmental Psychobiology, 58*(8), 958–967.

Maslow, A. H. (1962). *Towards a psychology of being.* Princetown, NJ: D. Van Nostrand.

Mau, M., Aaby, A., Klausen S. H., & Roessler, K. K. (2021). Are long-distance walks therapeutic? A systematic scoping review of the conceptualization of long-distance walking and its relation to mental health. *International Journal of Environmental Research and Public Health, 18*, 7741.

Mau, M., Klausen, S., & Roessler, K. (2023). Becoming a person: How long-distance walking can lead to personal growth – A cultural and health-related approach. *New Ideas in Psychology, 68*. Elsevier.

May, R. (1953). *Man's search for himself.* New York: W. W. Norton & Company.

Murakami, H. (2009). *What I talk about when I talk about running.* London: Vintage Press.

Nietzsche, F. (1889). *Twilight of the idols, or how to philosophize with a hammer.* Leipzig, Germany: Verlag von C. G. Naumann.

Ogden, P., Minton, K., & Pain, C. (2006). *Trauma and the body: A sensorimotor approach to psychotherapy.* New York: W.W. Norton and Company.

Oppezzo, M., & Schwartz, D. L. (2014). Give your ideas some legs: The positive effect of walking on creative thinking. *Journal of Experimental Psychology: Learning, Memory, and Cognition, 40*(4), 1142–1152.

Rogers, C. (1951). *Client-centred therapy.* Boston, MA: Houghton Mifflin.

Rousseau, J. (1891). *The confessions.* London: David Stott.

Van der Kolk, B. (2015). *The body keeps the score: Mind, brain and body in the transformation of trauma.* London: Penguin.

Postcards from the playroom

I recall being on placement, in the early days of my play therapy training, and working with a young boy who must have been around 7 or 8 years old. He was in long-term foster care, placed with a very loving family, but facing a great deal of uncertainty around his longer-term permanent future. The family were reluctant to formally adopt him, for fear that they would lose their current level of professional support and I believe that at the time this was a very real anxiety held by many foster carers. The consequence, for this child, was an ongoing state of 'permanent impermanence', never quite able to emotionally invest in the security of his future whilst also having to manage the complexities of family contact, which whilst important also unsettled the stability of his placement. He was a child whose both past and future was defined by troubled attachments and he found it hard, understandably, to form and maintain relationships.

I worked with him for about eight months, well beyond the timescale of my placement, due to his level of need. He was a gregarious, often quite feisty child and I liked him very much. Ultimately, our sessions together had to come to an end, as I was moving to another workplace. I recall our final session, talking about how hard it was to say goodbye and how I would miss our time together. We went through the many pictures and objects he had created over the months and that I had been storing safely for him, as he decided what he wanted to keep and what he wanted to leave behind. As the time came for the session to end, he said he had something for me and with half a smile handed me a crumpled piece of paper. I was touched and unravelled the paper to see two words written in big letters in red felt pen – 'fuck off'. I was still touched . . . I think. Endings are hard.

Chapter 6

Power, privilege and intersectionality

The politics of the playroom

Gardening leave

Recently, I undertook some work with a young adolescent. I will call him Ajay. Following his birth, Ajay spent some time in hospital due to medical complications before being placed in an orphanage and was then later adopted in the UK by a British couple, at the age of 2 years. At the time of referral, Ajay was exploring his transgender identity and had transitioned to identifying as a male, choosing to use the male personal pronoun – as used here. Ajay was experiencing a complex and challenging range of issues, including adolescence, identity, gender, sexuality, race, adoption and the impact of early developmental trauma. Following his referral, it was agreed that we would meet for six individual assessment sessions, followed by a review meeting to inform whether the sessions would continue longer-term.

Ajay was an engaging, sensitive, articulate young person, shy and somewhat introverted but with a sharp sense of humour and endearing personality; I liked him very much. Prior to the sessions beginning I felt a little anxious; working with adolescents is not without its challenges, and I wondered about the initial process of connection that can be so important in terms of establishing an ongoing therapeutic relationship. But as we progressed, my anxiety diminished; Ajay appeared to engage well in the process, and we seemed to have established the beginnings of a good relationship and I felt positive and hopeful about the potential for our ongoing work together.

In our sixth and final assessment session, Ajay was uncharacteristically quiet and it seemed as if something was troubling him. After a little exploration and gentle encouragement, he said that he had decided he did not want to meet with me for any more sessions and wanted to see a different therapist. He was apologetic and concerned about hurting my feelings, but after some reassurance that he need not worry about this and that it was alright for him to express whatever he felt, Ajay explained that he did not feel I was the right therapist for him, that I was 'too old' and that we had nothing in common. We had no shared interests, he added, and that there were things he felt he could not talk to me about. Whilst admiring his honesty, I was a little taken aback, there having been no indications of this in the preceding sessions. Or to put it more accurately, I had made the (false) assumption that Ajay

DOI: 10.4324/9781003352563-6

was actively and positively engaged in the sessions and would want to continue; a case of therapist arrogance perhaps, or the 'complacent competence' that I have discussed elsewhere in this book. Ajay had punctured both my assumptions and to a degree, my therapeutic pride, and whilst I would always be the first to acknowledge the things that at times make me a 'not good enough' therapist I have always felt that I am reasonably good at engaging with young people and had rarely experienced such a well-articulated rejection.

Shallow maybe, but I felt the need to push back a little and defend myself. 'So, what do you think some of my interests might be?' I wondered aloud. I wanted him to know that I was a writer, a hiker, a musician, that I played keyboards in a jazz-funk band – that actually, I might be quite interesting. Ajay came back without hesitation. 'Gardening, probably. Isn't that what most old people do?' Ouch, take that. But we laughed, and I made a mental note not to mention my allotment. Ajay was now warming to his theme. 'What is the name of the lady downstairs?' he asked. 'Oh, you mean Helen?' I replied. Helen was our receptionist; cool, spiky haircut, with a number of piercings and a tattoo. 'Yeah, she's alright. I like her . . . she's nice'. I was getting the picture; Ajay would rather work with Helen, our receptionist, than myself, his therapist. And whilst we could laugh and joke together about this, I was impressed by the extent to which Ajay, this quiet, shy young person, could express himself and feel empowered enough to state what he needed, to challenge my implicit assumptions and find a voice. And I told him so. Putting aside my slightly bruised therapist ego, for Ajay to experience a sense of personal agency, to say no, this is not what I want – *you* are not who I want – was perhaps the best outcome I could hope for. Therapist/client compatibility is important and in no uncertain terms, I had been told that I was too old, too white, too middle-class and too male. Lesson learned about intersectionality.

As a young, transgender, adopted person of colour, Ajay knew all about what it was like to feel marginalised, oppressed and disempowered. From an intersectional perspective, there was a complex and dynamic interrelationship of factors that contributed to his experience of oppression and his sense of feeling 'othered' by the majority group. To his credit, Ajay had managed to 'other' me, just for a moment, but perhaps he should not have needed to and that I should have been more mindful of my own implicit assumptions; of my white, privileged heteronormative status and the power differential in the therapy room. Ajay had been able to articulate his therapeutic needs and, in discussion with his parents, I was able to signpost them towards a potentially more appropriate therapist. But of course, many (most) children and young people are not able to do this, or might communicate their sense of disempowerment in other ways. I have thought much about power in the playroom; that however open, authentic and congruent we might seek to be as therapists, we inevitably carry into the playroom our own cultural baggage; our world view, our assumptions, our value system – and all the personal bias and prejudice that goes along with this. As a white, male, older therapist I also carry into the playroom my privilege and all the inherent power that this imbues; implicit and explicit, conscious and unconscious. Power and privilege will manifest itself through every aspect of the therapeutic process; our interactions, our reflections, our verbal and non-verbal communications, our session notes and our therapeutic formulations. To pretend otherwise is, I would suggest, an expression of power in itself.

In this chapter then, I aim to explore issues around my own experience as a white, middle-class, cisgendered male therapist and address issues of power and privilege and cultural oppression from the personal position of being within the dominant, majority 'group' that holds, or occupies, these implicit and explicit positions. I will also explore the notion of intersectionality and those multiple and dynamic factors that might contribute to experiences of either power or oppression. My central premise is that as play therapists, we need to be proactively cognisant about issues of intersectional oppression and, for myself as a white therapist, exercise a degree of cultural humility in this regard.

A note on language

I am acutely aware of the complexities around language and the words we use when describing the cultural world of people's lived experience. Words themselves carry with them a power, of inference, meaning and value, and whilst I am anxious about using the wrong words (and being judged for so doing) I do not want this anxiety to inhibit what I am wanting to say, however clumsily. Cultural and political discourse is an ever living, breathing, dynamic process of competing needs, wants and rights and within this, words, and the meaning of words, will inevitably change. This is particularly the case within the often rather febrile, hot-house of social media, which has accelerated the strength and intensity of cultural discourse, for better and worse. It can sometimes feel hard to keep up with terminology, and if I get the words wrong, I apologise. I hope it can be acknowledged that they are written with good intent.

Perspectives on power

Power relationships are complicated, often subtle and nuanced, often overt and direct. We can think about power within an interpersonal, relational context or on a wider socio-political level. Indeed, as I write this, thousands of far-right protesters are storming Brazil's supreme court and presidential palace in a brutal expression of perceived entitlement, an echo of the storming of the Capitol building in the US, on the 6th January 2022 – one group seeking to assert dominance over another. Power, and expressions thereof, are an inevitable part of the human condition on both a micro and macro level, and I would suggest that the two are not mutually exclusive. Power, like liquid, always finds a way; insidiously seeping through families, generations, systems, organisations and structures; coalescing and coagulating, pooled pockets of control and influence – benign or otherwise. Unlike liquid, the movement of power is not about finding a level; rather it relies – by definition – upon a sense of imbalance.

And as play therapists, we carry our own stories and narratives of power with us into the playroom – political, social and personal – and it is with some inevitability that these stories will again seep into our work with children and their families. As Fors (2018) suggests, even if we might like to believe so, we rarely find ourselves in positions of complete omnipotence or total powerlessness – 'we might embody generations of privilege and the associated questions of accountability and guilt . . . or we might embody the opposite: generations of cultural trauma. Most likely, we will in one or another way embody both' (2018: 10).

As a therapist, I am mindful of my own personal narratives around both power and authority, the two being interrelated but also distinct in meaning; power being more about the individual (or group) ability to control, direct or influence others whilst authority is predicated on a more perceived sense of legitimacy. Both hold a strong personal resonance. As written about elsewhere (Le Vay, 2022), my early childhood relationship with my father was complicated. Often highly critical and emotionally abusive (although not always) he wielded his power like a generational cast-off, a cathartic passing on of his own experience of paternal rule, driven much by the sporadic, inconsistent, scatter-gun impact of his own mental health challenges. I learned a lot about male power as a child. As a teenager, I was quietly rebellious; I dropped out of school, joined a band. I was anti-authoritarian and anti-establishment, rejecting my mother's religion but embracing her socialist firebrand politics. These early, formative experiences have all been a part of my ongoing personal narrative around power, authority and control, no doubt contributing to my decision to train as a therapist, and it is these personal stories and narratives that I carry with me into the playroom.

But also, of course, I carry with me my privilege and the associated power that comes with this. Power and privilege are inherent, inevitable, within all interpersonal interactions, including the therapeutic process and relationship. Much as there is a part of me that seeks to disavow myself of this privilege, to deny its presence or influence, this is simply a disingenuous pretence and it is, in itself, an act of privilege to be able to deny its existence, to be able to make that choice. It is not an option from a position of oppression. And for white therapists, there is a responsibility to acknowledge the dynamics of all that this brings. As Gil (2021) says,

> white privilege, or 'unearned power', inhabits our psyches whether it's consciously acknowledged or not. Play therapists and other mental health professionals have a responsibility to themselves and the profession to take stock of their attitudes and beliefs . . . anti-racist positions must be developed, planned, and articulated in thought and deed.
>
> (2021: 55)

It is not then, as Gil suggests, enough to simply acknowledge one's position of privilege, like some kind of easy, performative, self-aware confession. Rather, therapists need to act on this knowledge and awareness, to proactively address issue of power, social justice and oppression in such a way that it becomes embedded into practice. As Piper and Treyger (2010: 71) say, 'each therapist needs to wrestle with the question: are we agents of social change?'

This is not something that I always do particularly well, finding it all too easy to slip into a role of comfortable collusion, with both myself and others; to talk the talk, as the saying goes, but not walk the walk. Working within a predominantly white, wealthy, middle-class demographic, I can lose myself in mutual privilege, whilst overlooking other important aspects of power differentials. It should not have to take a young person like Ajay to jolt me back into self-awareness. At the point of his referral, I talked to his adoptive parents about how he might feel about working with a male therapist, but I did not consider fully enough other aspects of the power dynamic between us. And importantly, I did not have that discussion with Ajay himself until he raised it and whilst we did spend a lot of time exploring various aspects of his identity and his experience of discrimination and prejudice, I did not adequately address how he experienced our 'here and now' relationship in the room. This was a failing on my part, an example of my privileged short-sightedness and how, as Fors puts it, 'subtle cultural blindness may affect the therapeutic space and how innocent, unexplored benign prejudice and self-bias/self-centrism may be blind spots in the therapist that affect the transference, countertransference, and overall understanding of the (client)' (2018: 25).

I recall many years ago working with an Iraqi family who had sought asylum in the UK, after being trafficked across Europe. I was working for a service that undertook therapy and assessments with young people presenting with harmful sexual behaviour and the adolescent son of the family had been referred due to concerns about his inappropriate behaviour towards a peer. With colleagues, I met with the family several times, with an interpreter, and I met individually with the son for a number of sessions as part of the assessment of risk. Whilst we endeavoured to work as sensitively and thoughtfully as possible, I do not think, in retrospect, that we got anywhere near acknowledging the trauma, racism and oppression this family had experienced; being referred to a local authority child-protection service and all the potentially oppressive, statutory power that this wields. I am not sure how much the family understood about our service, about therapy, about the legal context of sexual behaviour and the criminal justice system. And I do not think we thought enough about oppression, social justice, trauma and the dynamics of western-centric white privilege and power. Looking back, I think we could have thought about this through a different lens and worked harder to empower the family, and it is with a certain degree of shame that I think as a team we could have done more. That said, we supported the family as best we could and completed a complicated assessment, hopefully with cultural sensitivity and competence, if not humility.

But the challenge – the need – is to be able to engage in open, honest and authentic conversations with clients about their (and our) experience of the therapeutic process, to explicitly address and acknowledge the issues of power and privilege, to bring it into conscious awareness so that it can be something known and named. For therapists, there is a danger of a collusion of avoidance, that certain issues and topics are avoided or skirted around due to the client's awareness, conscious or otherwise, that they are taboo or too challenging to address. As Piper and Treyger (2010) suggest, clients will often follow the lead of the therapist and if they sense a therapist does not want to address a particular topic, they will not address it themselves –

> perhaps the most important issue is the lack of and hesitancy of communication between therapists and their clients. Because therapists hold a position of power, they are responsible for using that power to broach pertinent topics that usually serve as a barrier within the relationship.
>
> (2010: 71)

Power in the playroom

Child-Centred Play Therapy (CCPT) needs then to be viewed and understood (and perhaps reappraised) within a framework of social justice and power dynamics. We need to think carefully about the principles, the core attitudinal conditions and language of CCPT within the ever-sharpening focus of culturally informed practice. As Cornelius-White (2016) suggests, the Rogerian (1951) principle of conditions of worth i.e. how external factors might determine how we value or measure our self-worth based on our ability to meet certain perceived or expected conditions, will also be informed by the experience of power, and differentials therein. So, for example, to experience a sense of social acceptance, a young person like Ajay might experience the need to conform to the cultural norm, creating an incongruent self-concept and consequent degree of 'internalised oppression' (Ceballos et al., 2021: 17). To his credit, and also no doubt to his cost, Ajay was able to express his authentic self, his trans-identity, and reduce his need to meet the perceived heteronormative conditions of worth. Indeed, part of his challenge towards me was an expression of this authenticity, a rejection of the cultural norm and dominant, majority values that I represented as an older, white, male, cisgendered therapist. From an intersectional perspective, this was just one aspect of Ajay's identity; as a young, adopted person of colour there are, of course, the added layers of oppression, discrimination and racism that he would be experiencing. Authenticity, for some, does not come without its risks.

Within the context of the core conditions of CCPT, we also talk about the principles of non-judgement and unconditional positive regard and again we need to be mindful of the conceptual language we use within a framework of power and privilege. It may be that we aspire towards these principles rather than accept them as a given. Is it possible, for example, to be truly non-judgemental as a therapist? Is not a therapeutic reflection or interpretation a form of clinical judgement? Our playing of a dramatic role? The formulations we make within our session notes? We are all making judgements, all of the time, about the children we work with and the families within which they live; we cannot free ourselves from implicit assumptions and unconscious bias, but we can strive to be more proactive and to bring to conscious awareness the potential enactment of privileging within the therapeutic process. In terms of unconditional positive regard – again, I would suggest there are always going to be conditions, implicit and unconscious, that affect the process; it is part of the transactional nature of power relations. So, within the context of power, privilege and social justice there is perhaps some reframing to do around how we understand and think about the principles and language of CCPT and how this translates into our clinical practice.

Fors (2021) proposes that power issues within the field of psychotherapy are evident in four specific areas; professional power, transferential power, socio-political power and bureaucratic power. This provides a helpful framework for thinking about power dynamics within the play therapy process. *Professional power* acknowledges that as therapists we hold status and authority; we get paid, hold records and make recommendations, liaise with other professionals and often work and report in conjunction with statutory and third sector organisations. However much we might aspire to be as open, explicit and transparent as possible, there will always be an overt imbalance of power, or as Fors puts it, an inherent asymmetry within the professional relationship. *Transferential power* lies within the therapeutic relationship and session content, the unconscious process, transference and client dependency – or indeed client/therapist interdependency. Children referred to play therapy are likely to have had negative, harmful and abusive experiences of adult power and been in positions of significant vulnerability, and it is with some inevitability that these dynamics will get played out within the therapeutic process. Whilst the person/child centred approach (Rogers, 1951; Axline, 1947) does much to acknowledge and address power relations within therapy – giving the child control, autonomy and responsibility, these dynamics will always, to a greater or lesser extent, be at play. I suggest that transferential power could also be thought about in terms of 'clinical power', the enactment of power within the session; the clinical material and the play process. This might include our interpretations, reflections and formulations – the way in which we might translate themes and hypothesise, however tentative. *Socio-political power* relates to wider, socio-normative, heterogenous phenomena; the impact of social, systemic and institutionalised issues such as gender, class and race and how these impact upon and affect the therapeutic process. This includes issues of power, privilege and oppression. The fourth area of power highlighted by Fors, *bureaucratic power*, relates to bureaucratic, controlling aspects of access to care and how 'subordinated groups are often at a relative disadvantage in obtaining treatment or social benefits' (2021: 248). This may be a result of institutionalised bias – embedded organisational prejudice and discrimination that creates inequality across social groups and that may impact upon access to care and, in this context, therapeutic support.

It is important that, as play therapists, we ask ourselves how these areas of power might inform, influence and impact upon the therapeutic process and relationship. At the point of access, referral or initial assessment, how has/is the family/child being affected by power dynamics and how might this be played out, both inside and outside of the playroom. Equally, what is our own relationship to these four domains?

How are we contributing to, or mitigating against, the dynamics of power that might lead to a family or child's experience of discrimination and oppression. Children have little or no choice about their referral for play therapy, as it is a decision made by adults and parents. They have little choice about when it begins and when it ends. We do our very best to act as therapeutic advocates, to facilitate a process that empowers children and gives them as much as possible a sense of responsibility, autonomy and control, but more often than not that is all it is – a sense of. Adults are objects of status and authority; on a fundamental level we are bigger than children, stronger, more powerful, occupy more space. And as said, for children who have experienced trauma and abuse, adults are frightening and dangerous. Power, and often in the case of trauma, male power, has particular connotations, meanings and associations for some children, so this might need to be considered very carefully.

I recall many years ago working with a young, 10-year-old girl who had experienced chronic, long-term sexual abuse, before being removed from her family and placed in care. I worked with her for several years and remember one particular session in which she instigated a game of catch with a ball. I wondered aloud if there were any rules to the game and she responded by asking whether she had to take her clothes off. This was her lived experience, her reality, of adult, male power, and is an example of the clinical, transferential power talked about earlier; those unconscious patterns of expectation that can get played out within the therapeutic relationship. I recall feeling profoundly shocked and saddened; this was a part of her story of male power, of abuse and entitlement – a terrible indictment of male privilege, in its worst form.

Some thoughts on intersectionality: a note to self

As Crenshaw (1991) suggests, intersectionality acknowledges that our interaction with the world is not solely based upon one aspect of our identity, but instead is complex, layered and multifaceted. Because the components of a person's identity interrelate, they are experienced simultaneously. Within the context of play therapy, a child or young person's experiences are shaped and influenced by aspects of their identity, for example their ethnicity, age, gender, sexuality, class and abilities. In this sense, someone might experience racism, transphobia, sexism or ageism collectively or individually at different times, in different environments and within a different context of interpersonal relationships. It is important that we acknowledge and recognise issues of intersectionality within our play therapy practice, along with the acceptance that some issues are more apparent, or visible, than others. As Mellenthin (2021) states,

> while it is easy to observe the overt gender, racial, or ethnic characteristics and makeup of a person, the more 'invisible' or less overt issues such as class, religion, sexuality, and socioeconomic status that are intertwined to create the intersectionality of how different systems of oppression and discrimination impact the client and their family, may be less easily identified.
>
> (2021: 139–149)

Equally, from a systemic perspective, it is important to explore with parents, adults and carers how a child or young person might be experiencing oppression, discrimination and powerlessness. Interestingly, in the example of Ajay, the adoptive parents were keen for me to continue – to 'push through' what they saw as his avoidance or resistance. There may well have been an aspect of this, but it was also important that they could hear, understand and acknowledge Ajay's voice and appreciate the potential areas of oppression that he might have been experiencing. As Ray (2021) says,

> acceptance of the parent's values serves as the basis for the parent to provide acceptance for their child. Just as in play therapy, as the parent feels understood and accepted, they are free to provide acceptance and understanding for their child.

(2021: 139–141)

Using a personal intersectional map such as that in Figure 6.1, it might be helpful to think about our identity alongside that of the child/young person, or perhaps imagined as overlayed on top of each other. Where are the points of confluence and divergence? What are the areas of privilege and oppression and how might we need to think about this within the context of the therapeutic process? Where might our blind spots be? What about our prejudice, bias and implicit assumptions/associations. See it perhaps as a kind of intersectional 'check-in'. Certainly, given my experience of working with young people like Ajay, it is an area of my practice of which I have become increasingly mindful.

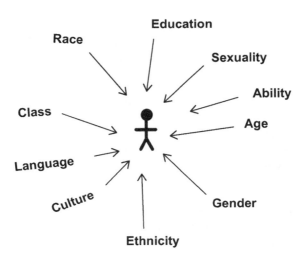

Figure 6.1 Intersectional Map

Source: image courtesy of Genesis Women's Shelter

Further to the idea of a kind of intersectional 'check in', I have developed something of a personal manifesto; some key principles to which I will seek to adhere and which might be helpful to share:

- I will endeavour to be aware of my power and privilege.
- I will endeavour to be aware of my personal bias and prejudice.
- There will be times when I am unaware of the above.
- Addressing issues of intersectionality can be uncomfortable. It is okay to be uncomfortable.
- Sometimes I get things wrong. Sometimes I fail. I would rather be a therapist who sometimes makes mistakes than a perfect therapist who is always right.
- I may not be the right therapist for some clients, or they might not be the right clients for me.
- I will endeavour to ask and listen to clients' personal stories of privilege and oppression.
- I will endeavour to challenge oppression and discrimination when and where I can.
- There will be times when I fail to challenge. I will reflect on why this is.
- I will endeavour to provide an affirming therapeutic environment for my clients.
- I will find out about what I do not know.
- I will endeavour to adhere to my organisation's ethical basis for good practice.
- I will endeavour to attend to issues of power and privilege both as a supervisor and a supervisee.
- I will continue to reflect upon this list.

Equally, it is important that these issues are addressed within training programmes. When teaching on an MA Play Therapy Programme, as part of the module I would facilitate a group discussion on power, privilege and intersectionality. It was a session that I always approached with some trepidation, knowing that it would touch upon personal aspects of the students lived experience and was a discussion likely to trigger strong feelings and potentially expose some of the inherent, inevitable intersectional fault lines within the training group. Often, the group discussion would become heated, rightly so, and centre around a competing 'hierarchy' of students' relative experiences of privilege, oppression and racism. Does being black trump being Jewish? Does being Jewish trump being disabled? Some might suggest that there is indeed a hierarchy of oppression, certainly racism, although it is a problematic concept and it might be more helpful to think about people's experiences being different but equal; specific and unique. Let us not fall into the privileging trap – all oppression is a bad thing.

But what I think was particularly helpful about these sessions is that the trainees began to think about their respective experiences of privilege and oppression in relationship to each other. Intersectionality is relational, by definition, and the group, in the safety of a training context, were able to begin to explore areas of difference and commonality; to hear each other's accounts of how they might have experienced power and privilege, to get a sense of each other's subjective reality and to have conversations about how this felt. Sometimes this was prickly and abrasive, as trainees rubbed up against each other – a testing of their differences. At other times it was deeply moving, as people took risks and shared stories with each other, some perhaps for the first time. As trainees and newly qualified therapists, they will be needing to have these kinds of conversations with their clients – with children, young people and their families. To have been able to explore and reflect upon aspects of their intersectional identity, to acknowledge or be challenged around areas of prejudice, assumption and discrimination is, I would suggest, an important process of developing self-awareness and personal insight and a critical part of what it means to be working as a therapist with vulnerable people.

Of course, there were issues about my role, status and privilege as a white, male lecturer (the irony does not escape me) and the institutionalised power of the academic organisation. Trainees rightly challenged aspects of the programme, the lack of diversity within the teaching staff, the somewhat white-centric nature of the resource literature and the need to diversify and decolonise the curriculum, not in any tokenistic, performative sense but rather a cultural, paradigm shift – a conceptual step-change around the nature of knowledge and a significant reappraisal of power relations and cultural perceptions within the context of the therapeutic teaching, and the theoretical underpinning of this teaching. If there is an expectation that trainees reflect upon aspects of power and privilege then there equally should be an expectation that the institutions responsible for the formulation and delivery of this training should also be open to the same process of self-examination. Suffice to say, this is work in progress. Further to this there are wider, systemic issues about the lack of cultural and gender diversity within the UK profession of play therapy, but that is perhaps a discussion for another day.

Uncovering, discovering and recovering

I subtitled this chapter 'the politics of the playroom', although I was not sure (and am still not sure) whether this is an appropriate term for what I have been aiming to explore in this discussion. Wikipedia (Politics, 2023) defines politics as 'the set of activities that are associated with making decisions in groups, or other forms of power relations among individuals'. We tend to think about politics in a wider context, in terms of organisations, agencies and institutions, and, of course, the state, but in relation to this chapter, I am drawn more to the OED's definition of politics as the 'principles relating to or inherent in a sphere of activity, especially when concerned with power and status'. I would suggest as therapists working with vulnerable populations, we have a responsibility to think about our 'sphere of activity', both the small and the big picture, the micro and the macro. Like the flowing ripples from a pebble thrown into a pond, we can picture the concentric circles of Bronfenbrenner's (1979) model of ecological systems, which views child development as a complex, dynamic interrelated system of relationships affected by, and impacted upon, the multiple layers of the wider environment; for example, family, school and beyond that, cultural values, belief systems, laws and socioeconomic factors. In this sense then, the personal is political and the political is personal. From a systemic perspective, we are not just working with the child in the room, but the multiple systems that are impacting upon their lives, just as from a psychodynamic perspective we are working not just with the child's present but the living, transferential and relational patterns of their past. Questions of power and privilege can clearly be thought about within this ecological context and so perhaps we can never quite escape the politics of the playroom and the systems of inequality that we are all subject to, in one way or another.

Issues of power and vulnerability lie at the very heart of our work as play therapists. It is, after all, what brings children to therapy. It is also, more often than not what has brought us to therapy; like two pebbles thrown into a pond, the ripples will overlap, intertwine and form new, intriguing patterns in the water. This shared experience of vulnerability is a veritable treasure trove of opportunity, a rich seam to mine. I recall once working with a young boy on the autistic spectrum – a quirky, inquisitive child, intrigued by the world around him. He had experienced a very troubled life of separations, traumatic medical interventions and consequent complex patterns of attachment. He walked cautiously into the playroom and noticed that there was something buried under the sand. Wondering what it might be, he got us both a small paintbrush and we proceed to lie down beside the sandtray, using our brushes to very slowly and gently brush away the sand. It was a meticulous process and we worked together at this activity for quite some time. As we worked, I said I felt a little like a palaeontologist, carefully uncovering the bones of some great prehistoric dinosaur. He said no, he was an archaeologist, discovering the remains of a lost city. So, there we were, the two of us, slowly, carefully, uncovering the past – our past, both his and mine. Our own truths, different but equal, in that moment. His early formative experiences had been of powerlessness and helplessness, frightening experiences over which he had no control. In that moment, the two of us lying on the floor carefully working away with our brushes, I felt a deep, empathic connection to this child as we each engaged in this small act of childhood remembrance.

As Sachs (2020) says, all therapists want to empower their clients, but this does not come from 'sound advice, robust pep talks and inspirational sermons' (2020: 167). Instead, we need to find ways in which to join and connect with the child's experience; to enable them to discover, uncover, whatever it is they need to – to step into their world, whatever this might look like. Sachs continues –

> it is in allowing and encouraging our (clients) to lead us into their shadows, accompanying them into to the darkness and joining them in being temporarily carried away by it, that the (client's) power, and the therapist's power to empower the client, are more reliably discovered.
>
> (2020: 167)

References

Axline, V. A. (1947). *Play therapy*. London: Churchill Livingstone.

Bronfenbrenner, U. (1979). *The ecology of human development: Experiments by nature and design*. Cambridge, MA: Harvard University Press.

Ceballos, P., Post, P., & Rodriguez, M. (2021). *Practicing child-centred play therapy from a multicultural and social justice framework*. In E. Gil & A. Drewes (Eds.), *Cultural issues in play therapy* (2nd Edition). New York: Guilford Press.

Cornelius-White, J. H. (2016). *Person-centred approached for counsellors*. Thousand Oaks, CA: Sage Publications.

Crenshaw, K. (1991). Mapping the margins: Intersectionality, identity politics, and violence against women of color. *Stanford Law Review*, *43*(6), 1241–1299.

Fors, M. (2018). *A grammar of power in psychotherapy: Exploring the dynamics of privilege*. Washington, DC: American Psychological Association.

Fors, M. (2021). Power dynamics in the clinical situation: A confluence of perspectives. *Contemporary Psychoanalysis*, *57*(2), 242–269. Taylor and Francis.

Gil, E. (2021). White privilege, anti-racism and promoting positive change in play therapy. In E. Gil & A. Drewes (Eds.), *Cultural issues in play therapy* (2nd Edition). New York: Guilford Press.

Le Vay, D. (2022). The child is the father of the man: Paternal patterns of countertransference and empathy. In D. Le Vay & E. Cuschieri (Eds.), *Personal process in child-centred play therapy*. London: Routledge.

Mellenthin, C. (2021). How do you address issues of intersectionality in your practice. In R. J. Grant, J. Stone, & C. Mellenthin (Eds.), *Play therapy theories and perspectives*. New York: Routledge.

Piper, J., & Treyger, S. (2010). Power, privilege, and ethics. In L. Hecker (Ed.), *Ethics and professional issues in couple and family therapy* (pp. 71–87). London: Routledge/Taylor & Francis Group.

Politics (2023). *Wikipedia*. https://en.wikipedia.org/wiki/Politics (accessed on 3rd June 2023).

Ray, D. (2021). How do you address issues of intersectionality in your practice. In R. J. Grant, J. Stone, & C. Mellenthin (Eds.), *Play therapy theories and perspectives*. New York: Routledge.

Rogers, C. R. (1951). *Client-centred therapy*. Boston, MA: Houghton Mifflin.

Sachs, B. E. (2020). *The good enough therapist: Futility, failure, and forgiveness in treatment*. New York: Routledge.

Postcards from the playroom

For many years I worked with children and young people with problematic and harmful sexual behaviour. These were children with invariably very traumatic histories of neglect and abuse, many of them in care with complex and troubled attachment histories. I worked with one young boy, who often needed to go to the toilet during his session. As with all children, I would walk with him to the toilet and then wait outside, occasionally calling through the closed door to check that he was okay. As a play therapist, I have spent an inordinate amount of time hanging around outside toilets; not always a great look and one that has often required some explanation. This particular toilet was located on the floor below ours and was shared by the social work team who occupied that floor.

He finished after some time and as it was time to finish our session he was collected and taken home. Later, when I was back in my office, I got a call from our admin officer who said that she had been contacted by the team downstairs who had asked that someone come down and 'sort out their toilet'. With some trepidation, I went down to check and found that the child had smeared faeces all over the walls and floor of the toilet – quite an impressive feat in such a relatively short time. I spent the next twenty minutes cleaning, wiping, scrubbing the child's excrement from the walls, floor and various nooks and crannies that he had very creatively managed to get it into. I would like to think there was something deeply significant or symbolic about this process, as I scrubbed away at the messy, shitty feelings of this child's internal world; that this was an important communication of some kind. But at the time it did not feel like it. It simply felt horrible, my capacity for empathy challenged by feelings of intolerance and disgust. Perhaps that was the symbolism.

Chapter 7

A postcard from the edge

Reflections on liminality and the role of play as a response to the Covid-19 pandemic

Introduction

On the 19th March 2020, my partner and I were on a plane from New Zealand to the United Kingdom, flying into the very epicentre of the global pandemic as we sought to return home and be reunited with our daughter, the world rapidly closing in around us. We flew around a changed and changing planet, sealed tightly within the metalled capsule of our Airbus 380, caught between time and space, reflecting both upon what lay ahead and what we had left behind. It was an abstract, surreal experience. We felt anxious and subdued but also becalmed, the soporific effect of the long-distance flight tricking us into a dreamy, dissociative state of mental absence that belied the stark reality of our situation. We were caught, both literally and psychologically, in the transitional twilight world of the 'in-between'.

It is hard to begin this discussion on liminality without some acknowledgement of the impact of the Covid-19 pandemic, itself a global crisis event and a transitionary phenomenon that has had long-lasting implications and consequences in relation to our experience of space and the meaning that this holds for us, from both a physical and psychological perspective. I will begin this chapter then with some reflections upon how we might view the experience of the pandemic through a liminal lens and the clinical implications this has had upon our practice, in terms of negotiating the therapeutic space. I will then go on to briefly discuss liminality within a context of recent socio-political challenges before exploring the more specific issue of play as a response to crisis, in particular the pandemic, and the notion of liminal space in relation to the play therapy process, exploring ideas of working on the threshold between comfort and discomfort, tolerating uncertainty and accessing creativity. This will include exploring the notion of therapeutic reverie and the 'in-between' spaces that as therapists we often find ourselves occupying as we move along a continuum between the conscious and unconscious.

Pandemic space

Humans are pro-social, attachment-orientated beings hard-wired for social connection, an evolutionary survival strategy borne out of the benefits of family/

DOI: 10.4324/9781003352563-7

group living – providing safe, protected environments in which we can grow and thrive. Complex levels of social interaction are an innate element of human development, from the infant through to the family and wider society. Social contact and connection are also integral to our experience of health and well-being, with research (Public Health England, 2018) indicating that loneliness increases the rate of premature mortality by 26%. The Covid-19 pandemic and resultant lockdown measures struck at the very core of our social identity, as enforced isolation and social distancing measures took hold. We were all confronted with the reality of physical proximity as a potential source of threat, leaving us having to re-evaluate the interpersonal nature of our interconnected lives. As social beings forced to stay apart, it was something of a relational paradox, one could say. An elderly neighbour, reflecting upon her memories of the Second World War in London, said that whilst the war was a traumatic experience, it was also defined by a sense of community spirit, of collaboration and connection – a sense of coming together in the face of adversity. Living through Covid, she said, was 'so much harder than the war'.

The pandemic had a profound impact upon everyone, and continues to do so, as its longer-term legacy continues to unfold, in terms of both physical/mental health and the ongoing political, social and economic implications that continue to play out – the rule of unintended consequences. With startling speed and impressive adaptability, there was a collective transition to a new, online world as we all grappled with a new vocabulary and new technology, a move from the physical to the virtual, and suddenly the strange 'here but not here' worlds of Zoom and Teams became the new normal; digital spaces and digitised faces. And after the periods of enforced lockdown, we emerged, blinking, into the dizzy, halogen glare of an altered world, having to find new ways to negotiate the space around us.

In a sense, the pandemic was all about transitions, as we found ourselves pushed to the very edge of what seemed manageable and tolerable; discovering new thresholds whilst never quite knowing what we were on the threshold of. There was no route map, it was unknown, uncharted territory, with no way of knowing how, if and when we would find a way through to the other side. As Rebecca Solnit says in *A Field Guide for Getting Lost*,

> the things we want are transformative, and we don't know or only think we know what is on the other side of that transformation . . . how do you go about finding these things that are in some ways about extending the boundaries of the self into unknown territory, about becoming someone else?
>
> (2006: 6)

In a sense, the pandemic has left us all feeling changed, feeling like someone else; an altered world and altered lives.

Derived from the Latin word 'limen', meaning threshold, liminality can be defined as a 'transitory, in-between state or space, which is characterized by indeterminacy, ambiguity, hybridity, potential for subversion and change' (Chakraborty,

2016: 146). It is often thought about in terms of temporal borders and ritual thresholds and associated with life-changing events, both on an individual and societal scale. Literature (Turner, 1969) characterises liminality by the qualities of disorientation and intermediacy and those ritualistic moments that mark periods of separation and reintegration, the transitory phase between before and after.

Certainly, the ritualistic liminal lens of anthropology can provide us with one way to understand the pandemic and as the Belgian folklorist Arnold van Gennep (2019) suggests, 'life itself means to separate and to be reunited, to change form and condition, to die and to be reborn. It is to act and to cease, to wait and to rest, and then to begin acting again, but in a different way' (2019: 189). Indeed, the pandemic found us having to act in all kinds of different ways, to inhabit new in-between spaces; the physically distanced 'two-metre' rule, the supermarket queue, gardens, parks and the confined perimeter zone of our one-hour exercise period. The social architecture of the public space was transformed overnight through a whole new language of civic mark-making; directional arrows, spaced standing places, lines not to be crossed – a kind of pandemic graffiti of social control literally writ large across pavements, walls and buildings. We all longed for the day when these cautionary images emblazoned across the concrete of our daily lives would simply become ironic, post-pandemic Banksy-esque art installation, more social commentary than lived reality. Perhaps that day has finally come. And beyond the physical was the metaphysical; that strange phenomenon of 'Covid time', a kind of temporal distortion that at once both squeezed and stretched our perceptions of the passing of days, months and years, another curious liminal space that marked our passage through the pandemic.

Van Gennep (2019), who first used the term liminality, saw the role of ritual (or the rite of passage) as a response to crises and change, be it on a personal, social or wider societal level, and defined this process as consisting of three discrete stages. Turner (1977a) goes on to describe these three specific stages as;

i)   Separation (from ordinary social life).
ii) Margin or limen – when the subjects of ritual fall into a limbo between their past and present modes of daily existence.
iii) Re-aggregation, when they are ritually returned to secular or mundane life – either at a higher level or in an altered state of consciousness or social being (1977a: 34).

It is then, a three-fold process; a separation or break from the familiar world, the reconstructive intermediate 'limen' of reflection and possibility, and a reintegration/incorporation into the world, informed by new insight and awareness. Interestingly, Turner viewed society as a process more than a static entity, a compound of successive phases of structure and anti-structure – an ongoing transformative, ritualistic process that he described as a 'realm of pure possibility whence novel configurations of ideas and relations may arise' (1977a). On a grander scale then, the concept of liminality can be applied to wider society as much as it can be to the individual, in the sense of periods of social crises that might be both destructive and constructive and lead to significant periods of social change, as we have seen during the course of the global pandemic.

The pandemic represented a transitional, experiential crisis, from the local to the global. Viewed through a ritual, anthropological lens and the stages of ritual passage described by van Gennep and Turner, we were all confronted with a disintegration or separation from the comfortable familiarity of ordinary life and a subsequent reintegration into what became colloquially known as the 'new normal'. And in-between was the liminal, intermediate space; an existential void in which we were neither here nor there – the day the earth stood still, to borrow the title of the rather prescient 1951 science-fiction film. Interestingly, films like The Day the Earth Stood Still and the plethora of other science-fiction B-movies coming out of Hollywood of the late 1940s and early 1950s, in the turbulent wake of the second-world war, were themselves thinly disguised allegories and metaphoric expressions of the cultural fears and anxieties of the time, for example fear of the Cold War, communism and nuclear annihilation. They were synonymous with external threat and fear of the 'unknown other' and as such could be seen as culturally playful responses to social anxiety. Similarly, the post-millennial trend of 'zombie apocalypse' films could perhaps also be viewed as an expression of infection-anxiety and the contemporary fears of the modern day, again an unknowing anticipation of what was to come. And just as life imitates art, with the advent of the global pandemic, science fiction became social reality, a happening so much outside of our realm of experience that, somewhat ironically, dystopian fiction became a significant cultural reference point for making sense of our experience.

The edge of reason

Liminality can also be thought about within a socio-political and economic context, particularly perhaps within the current, very polarised dynamics of cultural discourse that increasingly resorts to a process of 'othering' – acts of marginalisation and social displacement as a consequence of ever-competing needs and interests. We live in febrile times; Brexit, Covid, war in Ukraine, spiralling costs, dwindling resources and the increasingly evident impact of climate change, all of which I would suggest contribute to feelings of anxiety, fear and defensiveness. In the fight for safer ground, a kind of cultural post-colonisation one might say, people and groups who are not seen as fitting in with the normative, homogeneous needs of the 'majority' are pushed to the edges in often quite punitive acts of social thresholding, seen for example in the asylum policies of some governments. Covid-19 starkly exposed the intersectional, liminal fault lines of power and privilege, amplifying the reality of institutionalised racism, poverty and oppression. And consciously mining the fragile social seam of these fault lines, the recent insurgence of populist politics, which rather ironically sought to speak to the 'ordinary', has instead become something quite extraordinary; polarising families, communities and countries as cyberspace crackles with the deceit of politicians enthralled by their own power – take for example the 'partygate' scandal of Boris Johnson's government or Trump's cries of 'drain the swamp' as his own murky corruption was gradually exposed.

Gairola et al. (2021) have written about the phenomenon of 'liminal diasporas', which they define as 'subjective bodies in motion that are dangerously marked by difference, otherness, alterity, and precarity' (2021: 5). We have increasingly seen this in relation for example to issues of sexuality, gender and race and the rather politically divisive debates concerning the rights of refugees, asylum seekers or the transgender community. Individuals and groups, defined by their difference, are placed in positions of social precariousness, and find themselves played out in the battleground of competing needs, rights and identities. They are, in a liminal sense, neither in nor out, but instead forever caught somewhere in-between. As Turner states, the

> characteristics of liminality or of liminal *personae* are necessarily ambiguous, since this condition and these persons elude or slip through the network of classifications that normally locate states and positions in cultural space. Liminal entities are neither here nor there; they are betwixt and between the positions assigned and arrayed by law, custom, convention and ceremony.
>
> (1969: 95)

Like Covid-19, the climate emergency is dramatically evidencing this state of global precariousness, seen in the creation of new liminal diasporas as people are being increasingly forced into peripheral positions within this 'cultural space' – displaced populations, climate migration, homelessness, the closure of borders and colonisation of resources. As Dawson (2017) argues, 'as environmental disruptions proliferate across the globe, a condition well described as climate apartheid is becoming increasingly apparent. Climate apartheid encompasses the hardening of borders and restrictions on the movements of those affected by environmental and social disruptions' (2017: 194). Dawson's stark, perhaps contentious terminology, drawing an analogy between climate change and apartheid, raises again the notion of societal, intersectional fault lines wherein the climate emergency, like the pandemic, disproportionally impacts the more vulnerable and underprivileged (and generally non-white) communities. Often caught between borders, the refugee diaspora is not, by definition, afforded the migratory rights and normative privileges held by the passport wielding, cosmopolitan citizens of the free world. Be it climate change, Covid or international conflict, we are not in this together.

It could be suggested that the act of displacement often comes from a place of fear, or from something that cannot be understood, a kind of societal act of mass projection, homogenic fear perhaps, in which the intolerable anxiety engendered by the unknown is pushed away to the liminal edges, beyond thought or reason. If the reaction to perceived threat is a process of 'othering', be it individual, social or political, the challenge then, to bring this discussion back to therapy and the role of play, is how to facilitate a process of connection, collaboration and social engagement.

From the social to the biological, there is perhaps an analogy to be drawn here with neuroscience, for example with Porges' (2017) Polyvagal Theory, which suggests that social connectedness is synonymous with our bodily, felt experience of safety in proximity with another. The socially engaged pathway of the parasympathetic nervous system, the 'vagal brake', as Porges puts it, promotes those behaviours directed towards social connection and engagement and facilitates feelings of trust and safety as opposed to the more defensive mobilisation of the fight and flight response. In this sense, the creation of liminal diasporas, the pushing away of perceived threat, and the very split, polarised nature of so much of our contemporary social discourse could be seen as a socially mobilised fight and flight reaction, driven more by limbic, thalamic fear than reflective thought and reason. This, incidentally, is the populist power of 'dog whistle' politics, coded messaging aimed to appeal or pander to the fears of particular groups, aimed to disrupt and polarise rather than unify and connect. In essence then, Porges' Polyvagal Theory is about safety and connection and this is what lies at the beating heart of the therapeutic relationship. If as therapists we can help to minimise feelings of threat we can contribute, in our own small way, to a more connected, socially engaged society. And of course, the beginning of social engagement lies in play.

Playful responses to serious times

The pandemic was clearly a time of intense stress and anxiety. It was a dynamic period of change and uncertainty that affected people (and continues to do so) in many ways. Whilst being a global phenomenon, people's responses were unique and individual, depending on many complex factors, related for example to emotional resilience, social connectedness and the socio/political/economic impact of issues around institutionalised privilege, oppression and inequality (for example, housing and poverty) that saw some communities more vulnerable to the impact of Covid than others. In this sense, it is not possible to generalise the psychological impact of the pandemic across communities, but that said, anxiety and distress are natural responses to the threat that it presented and will have led to a range of coping strategies, some more effective than others. What was striking however, was the remarkable range of creative, inventive, spontaneous and fundamentally playful responses to the pandemic, an expression of social resilience in the face of great adversity.

Research (Hess & Bundy, 2003; Magnuson & Barnett, 2013) has suggested that both for young people and adults, play can be a significant contributory factor towards coping with stress. This includes the influence of playfulness upon the cognitive appraisal and evaluation of stressful events, the mediation and interpretation of stressful experiences and the role that playfulness might have in 'reframing stressful situations in a way that facilitates flexibility, reduces perceived stress, and improves resilience' (Barnett, 2007). The reframing of experience can be an important aspect of mitigating the impact of trauma. As social beings, we have a natural inclination towards the storying of experience, the co-construction of coherent, shared narratives that can help us to create a sense of meaning and context around challenging life events, and play can be an important part of this process. Research by Bundy (1993) also indicated that higher levels of playfulness resulted in greater levels of flexibility when dealing with challenging life events, supporting the notion that play and playfulness acts as a mitigating factor in coping with stress and anxiety.

An interesting research study by Clifford et al. (2022), which drew upon a range of measures to test links between self-efficacy, helplessness and playfulness during the Covid-19 pandemic, concluded that playful individuals (as identified by both themselves and others) had lower perceptions of stress and used a greater range of coping strategies to lessen their levels of stress. The research concluded that their findings were 'consistent with prior research that shows that playful individuals tend to use beneficial, adaptive, and stressor-focused coping strategies while less playful individuals tend to rely on negative, avoidant, escape-oriented, maladaptive strategies' (2022: 7).

The suggestion then, within this research, is that play is a valuable coping resource and for many helped to mitigate the very stressful impact of living through periods of enforced lockdown. Of note is that higher levels of playfulness were related to higher levels of perceived self-efficacy and that lower levels of playfulness related to higher levels of perceived helplessness. In other words, a sense of control and self-agency are important contributory factors towards the ability to cope with uncertainty and anxiety. There are parallels to be drawn here with play therapy. Children referred for therapy have generally experienced very little control over traumatic life events and as play therapists, we know that play can help children to feel empowered and enable them to develop a sense of self-efficacy and autonomy (Fall, 2010), and it is interesting to see this reflected in research around the role of play as a response to the pandemic.

The aforementioned findings also link to what we know from early behavioural research (Maier & Seligman, 1976) around the phenomena of learned helplessness, in which a repeated experience of a stressful situation, over which there is initially no escape or control, can lead to ongoing, persistent feelings of helplessness through being unable to affect the outcome of a situation, even when opportunities for change become available. In this sense, people have 'learned' that they are helpless, leading to potential feelings of anxiety and depression. Research and literature have made links between learned helplessness and the traumatic shock of the pandemic, and within this context it is encouraging to see subsequent research that supports the role of play as a way of counteracting feelings of helplessness, creating an alternate picture of hope and optimism and reinforcing what we intuitively know as play therapists i.e. that play is intrinsically therapeutic and healing.

It is important then, as suggested by the preceding, that we hold on to the centrality of play in providing a healthy, creative and imaginative counterpoint to some of the more existential challenges that seek to impinge upon our daily lives, be it Covid or otherwise. To respond through play is to creatively engage with the world and with one another and indeed, to play is a fundamental part of the human condition. As Winnicott reminds us, 'it is in playing and only in playing that the individual child or adult is able to be creative and to use the whole personality, and it is only in being creative that the individual discovers the self' (1971: 54). To return to the liminal theme of this chapter, the very socially fragmented impact of the pandemic forced us all into an anxious state of social limbo, treading water as we sought to keep our heads above the crashing waves, and perhaps it was partly the creativity of play and playfulness that helped us discover, or rediscover, both ourselves and each other, to reconnect and find a way forward.

Ackerman described play as a 'refuge from ordinary life, a sanctuary of the mind, where one is exempt from life's customs, methods and decrees' (1996: 6). The pandemic was clearly a time of refuge, both enforced and voluntary, and I think for many, play did indeed create a place of sanctuary – a creative response to a crisis that often threatened to overwhelm. Reflecting on my personal experience of going through lockdown with my family, it seemed that play and creativity were important aspects of our coping process. We walked, read, wrote, painted, played music and games, and even created strange, artistic structures in our garden, made from chicken wire, branches and leaves – probably for no other reason than keeping us playfully connected with each other. We were anxious, at times afraid, and at other times bored and restless. Perhaps, in its own way, our expressions of playful creativity were a response to this anxiety, a form of sublimation as an emotional/psychological defence. But it is also important to recognise, to borrow from Maslow hierarchy of needs (1943), that the capacity for playfulness and creativity is dependent upon the initial meeting of our primary physiological and safety needs i.e. shelter, food, warmth, sleep, stability and protection. For many, the experience of the pandemic would have challenged these very fundamental needs, let alone the more interpersonal need of belonging, characterised by the relational qualities of family, friendship, intimacy, trust and affection. For many families, struggling with issues of illness, grief, separation and the challenges of housing and income, the experience of the pandemic and lockdown was simply about survival and left little room for play.

But just as a seedling will push its way towards the sunlight, so creativity will tend to find a way. Indeed, the challenges of constraint and confinement can often provide fertile ground for the creative process, defined so much by its qualities of flexibility, adaptability and imaginative problem-solving. History has shown us that great creative achievements can occur under significant constraint (Stokes, 2005) and despite the acute challenges that the enforced lockdown restrictions brought to people's lives, I recall being struck by the wonderful sense of collective, creative inventiveness that emerged during the course of 2020, that strangest of years. This is supported in part by research by Hofreiter et al. (2021) that looked at the relationship between emotion, motivation and creativity during the Covid-19 lockdown, which suggested that there was a significant increase in creativity during this period.

Although not without its limitations, this research concluded that

> despite cultural differences and different subjective feelings toward the pandemic, results of this study show that we have one thing in common: when crises like the Covid-19 pandemic occur, we often turn to creativity to help us grow, give back, and get distracted.
>
> (2021: 13)

With the closure of theatres, cinemas, playgrounds and all non-essential gathering places, the home and street became the new pop-up performance space, with playful, spontaneous expressions of art and music being staged in the impromptu theatre spaces of front rooms, open windows, pavements, gardens and doorways. The meaning of space had to be renegotiated and new social thresholds explored.

Don't play what's there, play what is not there (Miles Davis)

The preceding quote from the seminal jazz trumpet player Miles Davis is a nod towards the more philosophical qualities of improvisational jazz and, as Davis also frequently talked about, the idea of 'playing' in the space between the notes. This is analogous to the concept of liminality, and as a jazz improviser myself, I can relate to the idea of playing on the threshold of what feels comfortable or familiar, often challenging convention and orthodoxy, and more often than not it is a place of great creativity and inspiration. Like Turner's (1977a) three-fold stage of liminality and ritual process, one of the defining qualities of improvised music is the dynamic of separation, reconstruction and reintegration; a falling apart and coming together with a magical sense of the unknown, somewhere in-between.

Childhood play, itself improvisational in nature, can also be thought about as the very definition of liminality. It takes place on the edges and in the margins of reality; under a table, on the stairs, in the corner, under a blanket or in a makeshift garden den. These are the borderless worlds of children's imagination, magically conjured manifestations of Winnicott's (1971) 'transitional space', the ill-defined, intermediate area of experience that exists somewhere between internal and external reality. Play bridges the space between the objective and the subjective, it is neither here nor there, inside or outside, but rather a transitional 'third space' in which fantasy and reality overlap. As well as physical space, play also occupies the liminal, intermediate space between the conscious and unconscious, bridged by the magical 'as if' qualities of symbolism and metaphor.

As well as a transitional space, play therapy can also be thought about as a ritual space. Ritual can be defined as a sequence of activity involving gestures, words, actions or objects, performed according to a set pattern. In this sense, there are many elements and aspects of ritual within the play therapy process. It takes place at a prescribed time and within a designated place and space. There are given patterns and conventions around beginnings and endings, creating a sense of contained repetition within which the child can experience a sense of safety and predictability. For example, meeting with the child and the walk to the playroom, the acknowledgement of time, the order of the words and language we might use, the giving of a five-minute notice before ending, the leaving of the therapy room and the clearing up afterwards, the writing of session notes. These are all part of the structure and analytic frame of therapy, the creation of both a physical and psychological space that feels known and safe. And within this the therapist and child will develop their own unique patterns of relating that provide a familiar shape and form to the session. And just as playfulness was an important part of our collective response to the pandemic, mitigating feelings of stress and anxiety, play therapy provided children with important opportunities to express and explore aspects of their own emotional responses to the experience.

For therapists, the pandemic-enforced transition into lockdown presented us with a complex range of clinical challenges for which there was little preparation. But as Turner also suggests, liminality is a space of possibility and opportunity, a threshold phase and condition of lived experience in 'which none of the rules and few of the experiences of previous existence have prepared us' (1992: 29), and in this sense Covid-19 was certainly a threshold event, facilitating a pragmatic and impressively adaptive transition to working online, the gaze of the camera replacing that of the therapist – as new liminal spaces were conjured up like magic out of the ether. Whilst an anxious and traumatic period, the pandemic demanded innovation by necessity, survival through resilience, alongside a revaluation of the rules of therapy, challenging the existing orthodoxy around boundaries, disclosure and the sanctity of the therapeutic space. A little like the jazz musician, this demanded aspects of improvisation, working on the edge of comfort; clinging on by our fingertips to what we knew and at times free-falling into new, unfamiliar modes of clinical practice. As Mastrogianakos (2022) stated, 'this is the essence of liminal learning: to come up with new ways to exist and move through the various spaces of place and mind and discover things about oneself that were not known or considered before' (2022: 241).

That said, as a play therapist I felt some resistance to the 'new ways' and especially cautious about working online; daunted by both the ethical challenges involved and my own sense of feeling insufficiently experienced in the medium to make such a transition. My training is in child-centred play therapy, a fundamentally relational process and whilst I was deeply impressed by the adaptability of those therapists who embraced the new world of 'teletherapy' with consummate pragmatism, I felt deeply uneasy about what seemed like a very different conceptual and theoretical therapeutic approach. Admittedly, this may also have been about my own rather introverted, luddite antithesis towards technology, but I also had significant concerns about the ethics, safety and confidentiality of working with children and young people online, and while therapy professions were able to consider this very carefully and thoughtfully, I made the decision to not undertake play therapy online, beyond some brief 'holding' sessions with ongoing clients with whom I was not able to meet during periods of lockdown.

Reflecting on this now, I wonder if some of my anxiety to working therapeutically online was also due to my many years of working with adolescent
and adult sexual offenders as well as children with sexually harmful behaviour.
Much of this offending behaviour took place online and as a consequence I
have developed a view of the internet as a rather dangerous space. It is said that
a little knowledge is a dangerous thing, but having through my work been part
of many police investigations into online abuse, it is more a case of too much
knowledge – leaving me with a rather bleak, tainted world view and it may well
be that this has translated into some of my unease about working with children
and adolescents online. The internet itself is something of a liminal space, a
digital threshold, offering versions of reality that need to be negotiated with
some care.

But I continued to teach and undertake clinical supervision online, along with
the limited clinical holding work during the periods of lockdown as mentioned
earlier. I recall one child with whom I had a series of brief fortnightly 'check-ins'
as a way of maintaining some continuity in our relationship throughout periods
when we were not able to meet in person. I agreed with the parents that the sessions take place in a neutral space, where they could be around, supporting the
child as and when necessary and joining us in any conversation that needed to be
had. The child often played out of view, or a disembodied hand or foot would flit
across the screen like some kind of UFO. For periods I would find myself looking
out into empty space, accompanied by distant sounds of family life, or a sibling
would walk by with a brief, defiant glance of envious curiosity. At times I did not
even know whether the child was there and who I was talking to. Sometimes we
played drawing games, or he showed me his collection of prehistoric monsters.
When he played off screen, I did my best to maintain contact through some kind of
verbal commentary, acutely conscious of my words being broadcast into the family home, like some kind of proxy visiting relative. At times it felt comfortable, at
other times intrusive and invasive, a window into the everyday theatre of family
life as impromptu conflicts would be played out, leaving me at times feeling more
family therapist than play therapist. But what I was most struck by was the liminal
quality of the experience, both in terms of the sense of spatial dislocation created
by the digital platform and the transitionary, in-between quality of the physical
space in the house.

Working online, the camera lens can take us into all kinds of spaces and places;
hallways, stairs, bedrooms, dining rooms, gardens. I was acutely aware of the
intense conflictual tension this way of working created in me; challenging, stretching and distorting the boundaries of therapeutic orthodoxy. Remote working is just
that; distanced, separated, removed and whilst I know many therapists who have
been able to adapt, adjust and integrate this way of working into their practice it is
something I have never quite been able to do. Relationships are about the spoken
and the unspoken. Attunement is about presence and connection, as much a felt,
embodied experience as it is a cognitive one. In essence, I find that the disconnect
of the online space challenges and compromises my capacity to hold true to the

core attitudinal conditions and principles of my practice as a child-centred therapist. As my computer rather ironically likes to remind me, sometimes my connection is unstable.

From despair to hope

I recently listened to a radio interview with Manni Coe and his brother Reuben, who has Down syndrome, talking about their book *brother. do. you. love me.* (2022). It is a moving story, poignantly describing their process of reconnection and recovery during the pandemic. Reuben, isolated in a care home during lockdown, sent a five-word text (the title of the book) to his brother Manni, who at the time was living in Spain. As Manni describes, Reuben's message left him with 'no choice' but to return to the UK and remove him from the care home (in an act playfully described as a 'bronap'), and retreat together for several months over lockdown in a cottage in the depths of the Dorset countryside, rebuilding their relationship, one small step at a time.

Reuben, as described by Manni, had experienced something of an emotional breakdown during his period of isolation in the care home. He had withdrawn into himself, become non-verbal and lost his capacity for playfulness and independence. Over the weeks, through a very gradual process of reconnection, they found their way out of the labyrinth, across the threshold and to a new, rekindled relationship – a process of separation, reconstruction and reintegration. But what I found most touching about this story was the strength of the brothers' response to the challenge of the pandemic, and that it was through reconnecting with his playful, creative imagination, within the context of a loving relationship, that Reuben found his way back to a meaningful life. It is a powerful message of hope, resilience . . . and play.

References

Ackerman, D. (1996). *Deep play*. New York: Vintage.
Barnett, L. A. (2007). The nature of playfulness in young adults. *Personality and individual differences, 43*(4), 949–958. Elsevier Science. NLD.
Bundy, A. (1993). Assessment of play and leisure: Delineation of the problem. *American Journal of Occupational Therapy, 47*, 217–222.
Chakraborty, A. R. (2016). *Liminality in post-colonial theory: A journey from Arnold van Gennep to Homi K. Bhabba*. Semantic Scholar. https://api.semanticscholar.org/CorpusID:39808309 (accessed on 23rd July 2023).
Clifford, C., Paulk, E., Lin, Q. et al. (2022). *Relationships among adult playfulness, stress, and coping during the COVID-19 pandemic*. Springer: Current Psychology.
Coe, M., & Coe, R. (2022). *Brother. do. you. love. me.* Beaminster, UK: Little Toller Books.
Dawson, Ashley. (2017). *Extreme cities: The peril and promise of urban life in the age of climate change*. London: Verso.
Fall, M. (2010). Increased self-efficacy: One reason for play therapy success. In N. Baggerly, D. Ray, & S. Bratton (Eds.), *Child-centered play therapy research: The evidence base for effective practice*. Hoboken, NJ: John Wiley & Sons.
Gairola, R. K., Courtis, S., & Flanagan, T. (2021). Liminal diasporas in the era of COVID-19. *Journal of Postcolonial Writing, 57*(1), 4–12. Taylor and Francis Online.

Hess, L. M., & Bundy, A. C. (2003). The association between playfulness and coping in adolescents. *Physical & Occupational Therapy in Pediatrics*, *23*(2), 5–17.

Hofreiter, S., Zhou, X., Tang, M., Werner, C. H., & Kaufman, J. C. (2021). COVID-19 lockdown and creativity: Exploring the role of emotions and motivation on creative activities from the Chinese and German perspectives. *Frontiers in Psychology*, *12*, 617967. https://doi.org/10.3389/fpsyg.2021.617967.

Magnuson, C. D., & Barnett, L. A. (2013). The playful advantage: How playfulness enhances coping with stress. *Leisure Sciences*, *35*(2), 129–144.

Maier, S. F., & Seligman, M. E. (1976). Learned helplessness: Theory and evidence. *Journal of Experimental Psychology: General*, *105*(1), 3–46.

Maslow, A. (1943). A theory of human motivation. *Psychological Review*, *50*(4), 370–396. https://doi.org/10.1037/h0054346.

Mastrogianakos, J. (2022). Covid 19: A liminal (transformative) experience. *International Journal of English Literature and Social Sciences*, *7*(5).

Porges, S. W. (2017). *The pocket guide to the polyvagal theory: The transformative power of feeling safe*. New York: W W Norton & Co.

Public Health England (2018). *Health matters: Community-centred approaches for health and wellbeing*. www.gov.uk/government/publications/health-matte rs-health-and-wellbeing-community-centred-approaches/health-matters-communitycentred-approaches-for-health-and-wellbeing (accessed on 13th April 2020).

Solnit, R. A. (2006). *A field guide to getting lost*. Edinburgh: Canongate Books.

Stokes, P. D. (2005). *Creativity from constraints: The psychology of breakthrough*. New York: Springer.

Turner, V. (1969). *The ritual process: Structure and antistructure*. Brunswick, NJ and London: Aldine Transaction.

Turner, V. (1977a). Frame, flow, and reflection: Ritual and drama as public liminality. In M. Benamou & C. Caramello (Eds.), *Performance in postmodern culture* (pp. 33–55). Madison, WI: Coda Press.

Turner, V. (1992). *Blazing the trail: Way marks in the exploration of symbols*. Tucson, AZ: University of Arizona Press.

Van Gennep, A. (2019). *The rites of passage* (2nd Edition). Chicago, IL: University of Chicago Press.

Winnicott, D. W. (1971). *Playing and reality* (pp. 1–156). London: Tavistock Publications.

Postcards from the playroom

Many years ago, I worked for an organisation whose therapy room was on the top floor of a very grand three-story Victorian building. One day there was a last-minute double-booking problem, with the play therapy room being used by someone else, so I managed to negotiate the use of another room on the same floor. My session was with a young adolescent, a likeable boy but something of a live wire, who kept me on my toes with his often quite testing behaviour. He lived in a children's home, having been placed in care some years ago. Outside the window of the room was a very inviting, flat area of roof with a fantastic view of the surrounding countryside, and towards the end of the session the boy said he wanted to climb out of the widow and sit on the roof. Whilst acknowledging his feeling and desired intention, I told him that this was not possible and reminded him of our agreement about keeping safe in the playroom. Hoping to redirect him, I said we could sit on the window seat and look out together. Undaunted, the boy said he was going to climb out of the window anyway and I said again that this was not okay, that it was not safe, and that if he chose to climb out of the window, I would need to end the session. This was one of the few times I have had to invoke the 'end of session' clause. The boy responded by saying he did not care about that and was still going to climb out.

With him being a quite stocky, well-built young person, I was beginning to anxiously weigh up my options, visualising the dramatic, plummeting demise of both child and career. I stated again that it was not okay for him to climb out of the window, that it was not safe, whilst attempting to manoeuvre myself between child and window to block his way. He was determined and I feared that the only way to stop him would be to physically restrain him, an extreme decision that could have serious ramifications. My options were quickly narrowing, and I recalled Rachel Pinney's book *Bobby* in which she talked about how children have an intrinsic sense of their own safety; potential accidents being caused mostly through adult intervention. So faced with the reality that this boy was either going to climb out of the window or need to be physically restrained from doing so, I chose a third way, stating that as it was my responsibility to see that he came to no harm, he could only climb out of the window if I went with him, that we could sit for a moment together outside on the roof and then we would need to come back in again.

And so it was that I found myself sitting on the roof of a three-story Victorian house with a child in care. We looked out at the view for a couple of minutes and then, ambition achieved, he was happy to climb back into the room and continue with the session. Needless to say, I never used that room again for a play therapy session and never again allowed a child to climb out of a window. Lesson learned.

Chapter 8

A view from the boundary

Introduction

I recently returned from a trip to Seville. In the evenings, my partner and I would often sit in our favourite square, the Plaza de San Lorenzo, have a glass of wine and immerse ourselves in the pleasant, gentle bustle of local life. As often seems the way in family orientated Spain, children played freely and happily in the square. Older children, in their national team's flame-red shirts, played football, their impromptu 'pitch' bordered by the cornered, ancient terracotta walls of the adjacent churches of San Lorenzo and Gran Poder. Sometimes younger children, having just discovered the excitement of walking, would toddle precariously into the action, always both welcomed and protected by their elder, temporary team-mates. Other children would run in giddy circles, scattering pigeons before them, or clamber around the time-greened, bronze statue of the baroque sculptor Juan de Mesa, standing proud at the plaza's centre. Periodically, the deep tonal bell of Gran Poder would ring out across the square, a timeless keeping of time, causing some curious children to pause momentarily and look around them as they sought the source of this sonorous intrusion.

It was interesting watching the children play. Some stayed close to their parents, who were perhaps sitting on a nearby bench or having a drink in the bar. They would make little excursions into the arena of the square, drawn towards the open space and the excited buzz of activity. But as if attached to their parents by invisible strands of elastic, they would soon reach a given, unsaid limit and be pulled back to safety, before setting off again on another exciting adventure. Whilst absorbed in their respective activity, both parent and child kept an intuitive sense of attention on each other, casual but cautious, mindful that the elastic did not stretch too far. Other children had much longer lengths of elastic, stretching in great orbital sweeps around the square, the gravitational forces of attachment much less apparent. Perhaps older, more secure, or in the reassuring presence of a guiding sibling, they explored the further reaches of San Lorenzo's playground plaza before returning to planet parent for a reassuring hug, drink or tempting bite of tapas. And other children seemingly had no elastic at all, somewhat adrift amongst the turbulent activity of the square. Each child had their limit, and some seemed to have no limit,

DOI: 10.4324/9781003352563-8

and watching them I imagined attachment as a theory of elasticity, stretch theory one could say; bungee babies, experimenting with risk and adventure – exploring the limits of what felt safe and secure. Sitting there I wondered about my own attachment relationships, and almost felt like tugging the invisible strand of elastic wrapped around my own waist, sending rippled wavelets back into the past to my own deceased parents, like some kind of temporal, coded semaphore. Would I get a reply? In a sense I do, as our early, formative attachment experiences lay down patterns for the present; my partner beside me, my daughter back home, my extended family. We all remain connected, one way or another.

At birth the umbilical cord is cut, establishing the baby's biological independence, but the invisible bonds of attachment continue to anchor the developing child to their parent, to differing degrees – some more securely held than others. And in essence, this is where our understanding of limits and boundaries begins, so evocatively illustrated by the contained, yet wonderfully permissive space of the Plaza de Lorenzo. For anyone wanting to experience attachment theory in action, you could do little better than sit in a Spanish square for a couple of hours of an early evening, a magical microcosm of human life.

To consider boundaries and limits within an attachment context means, by definition, to consider them also within a relational context. How, as play therapists, we apply boundaries and limits within the therapeutic relationship is a process that will be informed by both the child's and our own attachment history and early patterns of relating. Within an attachment context, therapy provides a secure, contained base from which the child can explore and, of course, this will be experienced differently by different children; testing, stretching, pushing, pulling, accepting, resisting, complying and defying, as they lean into those relational patterns that feel known and familiar, secure and insecure. Clearly, while certain boundaries and limits are accepted, set and applied as a given, for example the more static, temporal boundaries around session timing, frequency, place and duration, other boundaries will prove to be more dynamic in nature, revealing their need (and the child's need) as the relationship develops. As O'Sullivan and Ryan (2009) suggest,

> children receiving therapy may benefit from their therapist's deeper consideration of the attachment properties inherent in limit setting prior to and during interventions . . . limit setting seems to have a pivotal role in establishing therapists as children's secure base, containing their unmanageable feelings and enhancing their self-regulation and exploration of difficult thoughts and feelings.
> (2009: 230)

Within this chapter then, I will explore questions around boundaries and limits within play therapy. What exactly do we mean by boundaries and limits? How can we, or indeed is it even helpful to, place our understanding of boundaries within an attachment context? How does our understanding or application of therapeutic limits and boundaries change over the course of time and experience? Whilst boundaries and limits are seen as immovable, conceptual pillars of the therapeutic process, ideas around liminal flexibility will be discussed alongside an exploration of boundary thresholds within play therapy – raising potential challenges to the play therapy orthodoxy. This chapter will draw upon both my own personal developmental experience of limit-testing as well as exploring the idea of what it might mean to take 'therapeutic risks' within play therapy.

Lines in the sand

It is an interesting time to be writing about boundaries, in that we seem to be living within an increasingly polarised period of history; populism, culture wars, identity politics etc all relentlessly pushing the demands of competing voices raised against an ever divided and dividing society. The denigration of political discourse, courtesy of Trump, Johnson et al, inevitably spills over into social discourse, fuelled and amplified by the rather frothy, febrile nature of social media. The inclusive embrace of 'both/and' seems to be threatened by the divisive push towards 'either/or' and increasingly binary positions that do not allow for any thoughtful middle ground. Drawbridges are being pulled up and boundary lines drawn in the sand, not to be crossed. Pluralism and diversity feel increasingly challenged by the forces of separatism and isolationism, and to again place this within an attachment context, perhaps this is as much about a response to perceived threat and a fear of the 'other' in whatever form this might take. Like the children of the Plaza de San Lorenzo, a feeling of safety and security creates space for curiosity and openness, a willingness to explore, reach out and connect, whilst a feeling of threat or danger leads to retreat and withdrawal. Sadly, many politicians purposely play to this fear, thriving on a climate of anxiety and division as a means of holding onto power, effectively creating social silos; disconnected islands in a turbulent sea. And of course, boundaries can also be an expression of power and control, whether played out on the grand socio-political scale of border walls or immigration controls, or the punitive, distorted boundaries of an abusive parent.

I acknowledge that for a book of this nature I risk the accusation of being overly political, of even drawing my own lines in the sand, but I believe it is important. From an ecological, systemic perspective, one cannot separate the political, from the social, from the individual; they are connected, interrelated, each impacting upon the other, and when we think about boundaries, and the meaning of boundaries, I believe it is important that we think about them beyond the confines of the playroom. As therapists, how and where and if we hold the line is as much informed by our early, formative attachment experiences as it is by theory and practice and our ongoing experience of the social/political/cultural worlds in which we live.

As said, the application and adherence to boundaries is one of the key conceptual pillars of ethical therapeutic practice, but perhaps it is helpful to stop, pause and reflect for a moment upon our understanding of the meaning of therapeutic boundaries. Borders and boundaries, for better or worse, are a part of our lived experience, often denoting a point of separation or a metaphorical suggestion of power and control, a defining line that is put in place to limit or constrain, to hold back. In a literal sense, it is a marker that denotes what is out of bounds; one is either inside or outside; a fence, wall or territorial division. That said, I am reminded of the words of Rumi, the 13th century poet and scholar – 'out beyond ideas of wrongdoing and rightdoing, there is a field. I'll meet you there'. Like Rumi's field, a boundary might also symbolise a point of connection and meeting. It might be a stone cairn, a bridge, a river, a hedgerow, the sea shore – as much a place of growth and transition as it is of separation and division. Interestingly, Austin and Bergum (2006) suggested that the use of the term 'boundary' as a metaphor to describe, guide or conceptualise the ethical connection between therapist and client, is potentially problematic. As they state,

> a problem with the use of the boundary metaphor to envision the dimensions of therapeutic relationships is that the concept of a solid, rigid limit does not convey the softness of reality. Therapy situations are complex, more obscure and murky than clear and straightforward, coloured grey, not black and white. As comforting as concrete, predetermined distinctions are, they are not sufficient to guide professionals in all situations.
>
> (Austin and Bergum, 2006: 83)

So, whilst a boundary serves to delineate and define the edge of appropriate behaviours, helping us rule in and rule out what is appropriate, permissible and indeed ethical within the therapist/client relationship, it is also a point of contact, a place of meeting, which can communicate much about a child's needs, or their personal story of unmet need.

Boundaries are both intrapersonal and interpersonal. The realm of the intrapersonal is one of subjective reality, our internal, mental boundaries; the inner, intrapsychic division between what Freud termed the id, ego and superego. Freud (1975a, 1975b, 1975c, 1975d) suggested that the ego is a balance between the instinctual impulses of the id and the punitive morality of the superego, with the relative rigidity or fluidity of our intrapersonal boundaries being informed by our early life experiences and attachment relationships, potentially impacting upon our levels of impulse control i.e. how we manage, resist or succumb to the primal urges of the Freudian id. However much we may or may not choose to adhere to Freud's theory of the unconscious, the notion of internal, intrapersonal boundaries is important for therapists to consider. Our countertransference responses to the children that we are working with, our patterns of relating that we carry with us as part of our own unique, personal history, will inform how we respond to the boundary challenges that will inevitably emerge during the course of the therapeutic relationship. How 'thick' or 'thin' are these interior boundaries? What is the potential for them to become distorted or pulled out of shape? Do we apply our therapeutic boundaries differently to one child than we might another? The therapeutic relationship is a confluence, an entangled coming together, an ebb and flow of unconscious contact. Indeed, it is akin to the meeting of two flowing bodies of water, a merging of current, temperature, speed and depth and, of course, the boundary line between these bodies of water can become increasingly blurred and indistinct in the course of this alchemical mixing.

Interpersonal boundaries relate more to the realm of the external, the separation between self and other. This is more about our projected reality; those exterior, observable boundaries that govern our interpersonal relationships. From an attachment perspective, the nature of our interpersonal boundaries, and those of the children that we are working with, might communicate much about the relational context of family dynamics. Minuchin (1974), the eminent structural family therapist, viewed interpersonal boundaries within the context of the family structure, defining them as the invisible line of separation between the individual and the wider family sub-system. He envisioned boundaries as having varying degrees of permeability, from the rigid boundaries that allow very little communication between the individual and the wider family system, to the more diffuse, permeable and indistinct boundaries that can lead to a relational merging or enmeshment, seen for example in the impact or affect that the behavior of one family member can have on another. This quality of boundary permeability might communicate much about the nature of the child and family's patterns of attachment and is also likely to reveal itself within the dynamics of the therapeutic relationship.

Some theorists (Federn, 1952a; Hartmann, 1991) have conceptualised this idea of boundary permeability through the image of boundary thickness or thinness, a kind of continuum that sees at one end, boundary thickness, being characterised by a state of separateness and rigidity and at the other end, boundary thinness, being characterised more by a sense of relational merging and over-connectedness. This notion of boundary thickness or thinness, or that of both intra and interpersonal boundary stability (Lavering, 2014), is helpful in that it places our understanding of boundaries again within an attachment context. As therapists working with children who have experienced neglect, abuse or trauma, we are inevitably working with attachment and boundary issues, both intrapersonal and interpersonal. These are children whose experience of familial boundaries has been distorted, blurred and unpredictable; boundaries that on a psychological, emotional and physical level have been fundamentally breached, the lines continually being redrawn. Children will bring these experiences into therapy, play them out within the relationship, as, of course, we as therapists also bring our own patterns of relating into the playroom.

Some thoughts on risky play

Writing this chapter has led me to reflect upon my own childhood experience of boundaries and limits, and how this might have informed or influenced my practice as a therapist. As I have discussed elsewhere in this book, my own childhood was somewhat unorthodox, certainly bohemian. Being one of many children, growing up in the rambling wilds of the Sussex countryside, with parents who were often either absent, busy or pre-occupied, my own elastic, as it were, stretched far and wide; frayed and threadbare in places, but strong in others. My father's approach to limit setting was inconsistent, either non-existent or confusingly punitive, depending on his mood, which was always unpredictable. My mother, an emotionally generous, loving and caring woman, had what could best be described as a 'laissez faire' approach to parenting, more a matter of necessity than choice as she struggled to balance the competing demands of work, financial pressures and a growing family. Parental supervision was minimal, to the point of being non-existent, and perhaps like many large families there was a de-facto delegation of responsibility passed down the sibling line, a kind of parenting by proxy one might say. That said, as a young child I mostly felt secure; my patterns of attachment a rather complex, dynamic picture, held at times by my parents, my siblings and by a sense of place – the house, garden and surrounding countryside providing a secure base from which to explore.

And explore I did. In the absence of parental supervision, I had to find my own limits and in doing so took considerable risks. I fell out of trees, into lakes and rivers, played recklessly and wildly with my siblings, injured myself regularly – sometimes quite seriously – but ultimately revelled in the freedom to explore. In my own case, opportunities to engage in risky play may well have been taken to the extreme, more by default than design, but that said, the developmental benefits of outdoor risky play have been well documented. Reviews of research literature (Brussoni, Olsen et al., 2012) support the view that children have a natural propensity towards risky play and that, perhaps paradoxically, keeping children safe involves allowing them to take and manage risks. As play therapists, we do not need to argue the benefits and value of free, outdoor play for children; we know that through play children learn 'societal roles, norms, and values and develop physical and cognitive competencies, creativity, self-worth and efficacy' (2012: 3136) and that play is also key in enabling children to learn about decision-making and problem-solving alongside fundamental developmental qualities of control, resilience, regulation and the development and maintenance of peer relationships. Specifically, risk-taking play enables children – through experience and experimentation – to test their physical limits, develop critical skills around spatial awareness and perceptual motor capacity, and learn how to manage, avoid and adjust to potentially dangerous activities and environments.

Critically, it is through the experience of risk that children find where their limits lie, more a process of internal discovery than external imposition. I recall reading Rachel Pinney's seminal book *Bobby*, in which she describes the ground-breaking (if unorthodox) process of supporting a young autistic child's discovery and exploration of the outside world. Pinney concluded that an adult's sense of danger was a 'very unreliably yardstick' on which to judge that of a child's and writes that Bobby's sense of danger was 'uniquely his own and distinctly superior to that of most adults' (1983: 113). Pinney states that Bobby had an intrinsic sense of his own safety, whether it be crossing roads, climbing railings or negotiating the subways and buses of New York, and goes so far as to suggest that any potential accidents were caused only through adult intervention. In this sense, a child confidently traversing a seemingly precarious fallen tree, for example, is more likely to be unbalanced by the adult's anxious cry of 'watch out' or 'be careful'. That said, Bobby was accompanied at all times and was facilitated in safely exploring and testing his own limits. This is in contrast with my own free play as a child, with no adult accompaniment or supervision, but although I did experience many injuries along the way it is probably fair to say that these were mostly 'sibling induced', if I can put it like that, and it was rare that I got hurt whilst playing on my own.

So, just like the child traversing the precarious fallen tree, managing the inherent tensions between risk and safety is something of a balancing act. But it does seem clear that the experience of risk within play is important in the development of resilience, from a physical, emotional and psychological perspective. As Sandseter and Kennair (2011) suggest, risky play has an adaptive, evolutionary function in reducing anxiety around potentially fear-inducing stimuli, for example the fear of heights or water, through the natural and playfully repeated, progressive exposure to the given stimuli. Sandseter and Kennair argue that in the absence of such risky play opportunities, children may not develop their capacity to cope with fear-inducing situations, instead maintaining their fears which could translate into later life anxiety related disorders. In line with this, there is research (Beesdo et al., 2009) that suggests that parental over-protection is associated with increased rates of anxiety disorders in children and adolescents. It would seem then, that the health and developmental advantages of risky play are significant, although this is set against what often seems to be, within the context of play, a trend towards an increasingly risk adverse culture that limits children's access and opportunities to play of this nature. This is a trend that some (Eager & Little, 2011) have gone so far as to label as a 'Risk Deficit Disorder' and whilst this may be considered a rather pathologising overstatement it does highlight the potential threat that an overly excessive focus on safety can pose to healthy child development.

Nooks and crannies: risk in the playroom

Given my early childhood experiences of risky play, I am curious as to how this has informed my practice as a play therapist. I have always had a very high tolerance of the very messy, chaotic and sometimes risky edges of children's play; of allowing children to find their own limits within the bounds of physical and emotional safety and perhaps at times this has tipped into being overly permissive, but I would rather that than be overly restrictive. However, although often used interchangeably, it is important here to emphasise the distinction between limits and boundaries and what this might mean in terms of risk.

Limit setting is directed towards the management of the child's behaviour within the playroom. As Landreth (1991) states, limit setting is 'one of the most important aspects of play therapy and is also one of the most problematic' (1991: 209), adding that limit setting seems to be the single most challenging area for play therapists. For the trainee therapist, there might be a tendency to be uncertain or over-cautious in applying limits or conversely a tendency towards the over-application of limits, driven by an anxiety that can become more controlling than permissive. But limits are important in providing a containing structure for the development of the relationship and again, as Landreth states, 'without limits a relationship would have little value' (1991: 209). Limit setting then, in its most basic sense, refers to what a child can and cannot do in the playroom, and is integral to the establishment of a safe, contained, consistent and emotionally secure therapeutic space.

Boundaries, on the other hand, are relational and can be understood more within an interpersonal and intrapersonal context, being concerned with the parameters of personal, societal and cultural norms of behaviour. Within the context of the therapeutic relationship, boundaries define the appropriately expected and accepted level of physical and psychological proximity between therapist and child. Indeed, boundaries are the basis of sound ethical and moral conduct; ethical in relation to matters of jurisprudence and the professional frameworks and codes of practice within which we practice, and moral in relation to our own personal values and our commitment to the therapeutic principles of beneficence and non-maleficence. As discussed earlier, boundaries are also intrapersonal, in the sense of those more internal factors that might inform or influence a therapist's thoughts, feelings and behaviours, particularly in the sense of managing issues around impulse control and emotional regulation or our countertransference responses – perhaps played out through our sometimes narcissistic need to be liked, wanted or needed. Again, as previously stated, the respective 'thickness' or 'thinness' of our intrapersonal boundaries, their degree of relative rigidity or fluidity, is informed by our early, formative attachment experiences. Both child and therapist will bring the story of their lived intrapersonal history into the present moment of the interpersonal relationship.

So whilst, in terms of limits, I am very tolerant and permissive in my approach to managing the often very messy feelings (and behaviour) that a child will bring to therapy, I have always been very mindful about my attendance to the boundaries of the interpersonal relationship. It is, after all, the experience of distorted, enmeshed and often abusive interpersonal boundaries that has brought the child to therapy, and it is important that these dynamics do not get unhelpfully replayed. Children will often want to play out those interpersonal patterns of relating that feel known and familiar, testing the resilience and robustness of the therapeutic relationship. The challenges of interpersonal boundaries might then get played out within the unconscious process, patterns of transference and countertransference that trigger areas of unmet need for both child and therapist. Or it might be issues of confidentiality, self-disclosure, enmeshment or physical proximity.

In relation to risk in the playroom, this will look different depending on the context i.e. if it is concerned with either limits or boundaries. I have worked with children who have wanted to climb out of windows, climb on furniture, harm me or themselves. There is both the overt, conscious testing of limits and the more inadvertent, risky nature of children's play, for example a ball breaking a lightbulb or a child tripping and hurting themselves etc. Children who have grown up in family situations where there have been minimal or inconsistent limits will push to see where the limits lie – what it is they can and cannot do. After all, within CCPT we tell children that they can do almost anything they choose and naturally they will test this statement both to see if it is true and to test our capacity as therapists to hold, manage and contain these limits within the playroom. Personally, it is the behavioural limit testing that I have found more straightforward to manage, being more overt, explicit and visible. Taking my lead from Rachel Pinney, I have learned to trust children's sense of safety and manage my own anxiety in response to potential risk.

Managing the more amorphous, relational risks around boundary issues can be much more challenging as they are invariably caught up in the entangled space between the inter and intrapersonal. This might involve negotiating issues of confidentiality with young people who self-harm or express suicidal feelings; the risk of a young person disengaging or withdrawing if they feel their trust has been compromised. There are the relative risks or gains around self-disclosure and how this might impact the therapeutic process. Similarly, managing issues around proximity or physical contact, especially with children who have experienced trauma and abuse. I recall working with a severely traumatised girl who was very triggered around the issue of physical proximity and the paradoxical tension between wanting to be close but being afraid of being near, a legacy of disorganised attachment and her experience of adults as dangerous and unpredictable. If I sat too close to her or moved too quickly, she would become highly dissociative and dysregulated, so the challenge was in finding the optimal point of physical and emotional proximity – to know where her own boundary lines were drawn.

There are risks within the unconscious process; the dynamics of transference and countertransference that can distort our boundaries and pull them out of shape, for example the children who invoke strong maternal or paternal responses leading to over-involvement and a sense of relational merging. Or children who invoke our internalised critical parent and who we might want to distance by applying boundaries punitively. There are risks of interpretation and reflection; of saying the wrong thing or not saying anything at all. It could be suggested that much of the important work we do as play therapists takes place at the edge of what feels comfortable and tolerable, knowable and unknowable, within those liminal, transitional nooks and crannies of the therapeutic space. But of course, from an attachment perspective, children need to feel safe in order to explore and to find where these limits lie, and so there is a direct correlation between safety and risk, it is what brings children to therapy. Ultimately, play therapy is all about limits and boundaries; they are the field of contact, of both separation and meeting, the living skin of the therapeutic encounter, the containing embrace of Winnicott's (1958) 'good enough mother' –

loosely yet firmly encompassing arms that imperfectly protect from harm while holding a space of permission to experiment with a different way of being and doing in the world, including learning how to compensate for imperfect boundaries to create containment and safety for self.

(Rodgers, 2009: 52)

Crossings, transgressions and violations

Whilst boundaries and limits are a cornerstone of ethical practice, it is equally important that their application is not so rigid or laid down in concrete, as to diminish or detract from the natural humanity of the therapeutic encounter. In this sense, it could be suggested that there is a boundary/permissiveness continuum; that perhaps as we become more experienced and confident in our therapeutic practice and comfortable within a developing sense of our intuitive 'unconscious competence' (Broadwell, 1969), we are, like Rumi's field, more able to experience boundaries as a relational meeting place, rather than a border wall. In terms of a permissive continuum, we might apply our boundaries and limits differently to one child than we do another, rather than a 'blanket' approach to all children. This is partly about an understanding of the limit/boundary testing behaviour; what is the feeling beneath the behaviour and the need beneath the feeling. Is it an expression of attachment need or trauma or neurodiversity, or indeed something else? This permissiveness or boundary permeability might include a degree of what could be considered a boundary crossing or transgression, rule breaking even, challenging the prevailing play therapy orthodoxy and the unquestionable adherence to rules, limits and boundaries.

Of course, I say this with some care and caution and within a context that acknowledges the necessity of clear and safe boundaries as the basis for sound ethical practice. As Owen (1997) states, we can understand the concept of boundaries as referring to those expectations and requirements of therapists for 'appropriate behaviour that have been set by their professional body, their training and the professional literature, which explicitly or implicitly defines required and disallowed forms of behaviour' (1997: 163). But I would be equally cautious about the blanket, over-adherence to boundaries and limits that might prove detrimental to the therapeutic relationship. As Woskett (1999) argues, the ethical use of self within therapy can accommodate a developing and evolving understanding and management of boundaries. In this sense, 'boundary management may increasingly come to mean a reliance on internalised and intuitive holding structures that have less to do with observing externally set limits than with knowing oneself and what one is capable of containing and sustaining' (1999: 163).

It is important here to make the distinction between boundary crossings and boundary violations. To this end, Gutheil and Gabbard (1993) state that a boundary crossing is a deviation from conventional therapeutic activity that is harmless and non-exploitative and possibly even beneficial to the therapy itself. In contrast, a boundary violation is harmful and potentially abusive, both to the client and the therapy. In this sense it constitutes an exploitation of the client and an expression of therapist power and status. Further to this, Hartmann (1997) defined a boundary violation as an event or act that occurs whenever the therapist is responding to their own need and fails to act in the best interests of the client i.e. the therapist privileges their own needs over those of the client.

As discussed elsewhere in this book, the dynamics of power and privilege will always to some extent be at play within the therapeutic relationship and it is important to consider the potential role of boundaries in furthering or protecting the power, status and authority of the professional. Some theorists (Collier, 1987) have seen this as a function of patriarchy, highlighting the role of gender in the stipulation and conceptualisation of boundaries within the therapeutic relationship. Others (Rodgers, 2009) have suggested that the therapeutic limiting function of boundaries is more an expression of therapist fear and anxiety. Rodgers suggests that the intimate nature of the therapeutic relation requires, by definition, the therapist to enter into an intimate relationship with themselves, adding that this is a challenge that many are not prepared to meet – 'choosing rather the safety, comfort, and protection of formal and formularized boundaries' (2009: 52). As Rowan and Jacobs (2002) have stated,

> the fear in the therapist is of disorganisation of the self, or of the client, or of the relationship between them; and catastrophic expectations on the part of the therapist that make them restrict their work to what is safe and unexceptionable.
>
> (2002: 131)

In this sense, and rather paradoxically, the more common boundary violations might well be those of excessive distance rather than over-involvement (Lewin, 1994). Play therapy is relational, it is about contact and connection, and so we need to be mindful that we do not apply boundaries and limits in such a way as to create a wall that separates us from the child. If we do, they will either make every effort to climb over it or retreat and disconnect. Instead, effective boundaries should define a 'fluctuating, reasonably neutral, safe space that enables the dynamic, psychological interaction between therapist and patient to unfold' (Beauchamp, 1999).

Some boundary questions

The question of touch within play therapy has been much debated (Courtney & Nolan, 2017). We are invariably working with children whose boundaries have been fundamentally breached, emotionally, psychologically and sexually, through an abuse of adult power. As adult therapists we are also in a position of power and the child in a position of vulnerability. As a male therapist and having worked for many years with children presenting with harmful and problematic sexual behaviour, I am very cautious about touch, as much for my own safety as that of the child's. Conversely, these are children who can also feel untouchable, the palpable anxiety that surrounds them creating a sense of toxic fear around the act of physical contact. I have worked with children's homes and foster placements where there have been strict 'no touching' policies, and it is not hard to imagine the impact this will have upon a child's sense of shame, self-esteem and self-concept. Touch can be harmful and often has been for the children we work with, but it is also about human connection and it is important that we do not become so risk adverse, or driven by fear and anxiety, that we lose our natural capacity to respond humanely.

I would never instigate touch, certainly not without a child's consent, but the simple act of a handshake (or post-Covid, a fist bump), even with very young children, can be a playful way of engaging in a safe form of contact. I would never hug a child, although on many occasions I have been ambushed with a hug, catching me off guard, and whilst I might well try to redirect these approaches towards more appropriate forms of therapist/child contact, I also do not want to reinforce feelings of shame or rejection.

I once worked with a deeply neglected fostered child, a young boy, who became increasingly regressive in his play, as he revisited and replayed key developmental stages from his very early life. Over the weeks, he gradually stopped talking and started babbling like a pre-verbal infant and played out repeated scenes of being pulled out from various womb-like structures that he created from chairs, foam blocks and blankets. This culminated in one session when, as we sat side by side next to the sandtray, he sought to climb onto my lap, saying in his very little voice, 'now you have to borne me'. Normally, I would avoid physical contact at this level of intimacy, perhaps redirecting him towards cushions, blankets or a beanbag as a substitute, but this felt important, within the attachment context of his play, and so I allowed him to clamber onto my lap. He then proceeded to slide down between my legs, right into the sandtray, where he lay quiet for a few moments before letting out the primal, bellowing scream of a new-born infant. Over the subsequent weeks, he began to 'grow up' again, moving from crawling to walking and talking. On reflection, allowing this level of physical contact was certainly something of a boundary transgression and I wondered if I would have done the same had this been a girl – probably not. But it was what he needed to do and to have prevented or hindered this process through a rigid adherence to the application of boundaries would, in my view, have detrimentally impacted the therapeutic process and even felt unethical.

Therapy is a relationship, a human encounter, and as therapists we sometimes need to make intuitive decisions as to what feels therapeutically 'right' or 'appropriate'. To uniformly adhere to a set of therapy rules etched in concrete can diminish the human nature of our therapeutic field of contact. To build the walls even higher, as a way of protecting or distancing ourselves might not serve the therapeutic interests of the child. As Brown (1994) suggests, the unthinking compliance to concrete rules is not necessarily the way to promoting ethical practice. Rather, Brown believed that ethics need to be treated as a foundation for practice as opposed to an afterthought or something added on after the fact – 'it would seem that if ethical boundaries are entirely contingent on external constraints, there exists a serious problem. Ethical considerations must also come from within: Ethical relationships evolve from the enactment of ethical values by individual professionals' (Austin and Bergum, 2006).

The boy was finally placed with an adoptive family on the other side of the country. Many months later I was contacted by the adoptive parents to say that he had asked if I could visit. Normally, I would not have contact with children outside their sessions, but again this somehow felt instinctively right – for him to know that

I still existed and that our relationship remained intact, joined, in that powerful act of symbolic birthing. So I did travel several hundred miles to spend an afternoon with him, perhaps another boundary transgression. They lived on the coast and we spent time playing in the sand on the beach near their home, an evocative echo of our play therapy sessions together.

Similarly, taking the often very thorny issue of self-disclosure, there have been occasions when I have crossed the hallowed line and shared sometimes quite personal information about myself. For example, I recall working with a young adolescent with a learning disability whose father had died. Noting that I was 'quite old' he asked me if my own father was dead. I replied, yes, he is dead – like your own father – and that it is very difficult to lose a parent. We were able to join for a moment in our shared loss, to find a point of connection. To have batted this question back with a stock response would have felt incongruent and unhelpful. But again it is about context and meaning and in this case the use of self-disclosure as an intervention, even though in the moment I had little time to think about it, simply felt right. With other children I may be much more careful about what I disclose. But interestingly, as time has gone on, I have generally felt more comfortable with sharing aspects of my own experience, self-disclosure and the use of self. Perhaps I am more relaxed about it or prepared to take more risks, or indeed have allowed my boundaries to become more permeable.

For many years I worked within a therapy service for children in the care system, the therapy rooms being located on the site of a residential children's home. Invariably, these were children and adolescents who had experienced high levels of trauma and abuse and who had been through multiple family placements, foster and adoptive placements that had broken down, ultimately compounding the narrative of the child who is unplaceable and facing a future in long-term residential care. These were young people with deeply complex, disturbed attachment histories, their narrative identity informed by powerful stories of loss and rejection. In terms of therapy, issues of engagement and trust were key and both boundaries and limits were tested to the extreme. Often, the intimacy of the playroom felt too intense, and it was not uncommon for me to be conducting sessions in the extensive grounds of the children's home.

Sometimes we climbed trees and sat amongst the branches. Sometimes we walked around the pond, looking for frogspawn or newts. Sometimes we played football. Sometimes we made dens together. At all times I had to manage and hold a degree of risk and that exciting quality of the unknown afforded by the outside world. The relationship took us beyond the bounds of the playroom, challenging the rules, limits and boundaries of the conventional play therapy orthodoxy of my training. It was a question of containment, enabling the young person to feel safe and held and beyond the four walls of the playroom and ultimately it was the attachment relationship that provided the secure base from which we could explore. As said earlier, for many of these young people, the challenge was one of proximity, both physical and emotional, and the paradoxical tension of wanting to be close but not wanting to be near.

My sense was that for many of these young people, with their complex attachment histories, being in the playroom intensified and magnified these tensions, leaving them with little recourse but to challenge and push the limits even further. Being outside, albeit being beyond conventional practice, made these issues of proximity feel more manageable, the tensions absorbed, held and contained by the non-judgemental, calming essence of the natural world around us. The site had a playing field, and like Rumi's field, it was a place of meeting, a place 'beyond ideas of wrongdoing and rightdoing'. Perhaps as Austin and Bergum suggest, we can 'move beyond our traditional metaphor of boundary as the dominant means of structuring the way we think about and respond to issues of therapist-client relationships' (2006: 91). It might be a field, a tree, a pond or even our favourite square in Seville, the Plaza de San Lorenzo, where children playfully explore their limits, tugging at the invisible strands of elastic that bond them to their parents. Boundaries and limits are about contact and connection, an expression of unmet need, as much as they are about separation. Let us not build more walls; there are more than enough of these in our world as it is.

References

Austin, W., & Bergum, V. (2006). A re-visioning of boundaries in professional helping relationships: Exploring other metaphors. *Ethics & Behavior*, *16*(2), 77–94.

Beauchamp, T. L. (1999). The philosophical basis of psychiatric ethics. In S. Bloch, P. Chodoff, & S. A. Green (Eds.), *Psychiatric ethics* (3rd Edition, pp. 25–48). Oxford: Oxford University Press.

Beesdo, K., Knappe, S., & Pine, D. S. (2009). Anxiety and anxiety disorders in children and adolescents: Developmental issues and implications for DSM-V. *Psychiatric Clinics of North America*, *32*, 483–524.

Broadwell, M. (1969). *Teaching for learning (XVI)*. wordsfitlyspoken.org. The Gospel Guardian (accessed on 11th May 2018).

Brown, L. S. (1994). Concrete boundaries and the problem of literal-mindedness: A response to Lazarus. *Ethics & Behavior*, *4*, 275–281.

Brussoni, M., Olsen, L., Pike, I., & Sleet, D. (2012). Risky play and children's safety: Balancing priorities for optimal child development. *International Journal of Environment Research and Public Health*, *9*, 3134–3148. https://doi.org10.3390/ijerph9093134.

Collier, H. V. (1987). The differing self: Women as psychotherapists. In M. Baldwin & V. Satir (Eds.), *The use of self in therapy* (pp. 53–60). New York: Haworth.

Courtney, J., & Nolan, R. (Eds.) (2017). *Touch in child counseling and play therapy: An ethical and clinical guide*. Abingdon, UK: Routledge.

Eager, D., & Little, H. (2011). *Risk deficit disorder*. In Proceeding of IPWEA International Public Works Conference. Melbourne.

Federn, P. (1952a). The ego as subject and object in narcissism. In E. Weiss (Ed.), *Ego psychology and the psychoses* (pp. 283–322). New York: Basic Books.

Freud, S. (1975a). Consciousness and what is unconscious. In J. Strachey (Ed. and Trans.), *The standard edition of the complete psychological works of Sigmund Freud* (Vol. 19, pp. 13–18). London: Hogarth Press. (Original work published 1923).

Freud, S. (1975b). The ego and the id. In J. Strachey (Ed. and Trans.), *The standard edition of the complete psychological works of Sigmund Freud* (Vol. 19, pp. 19–27). London: Hogarth Press. (Original work published 1923).

Freud, S. (1975c). The ego and the super-ego. In J. Strachey (Ed. and Trans.), *The standard edition of the complete psychological works of Sigmund Freud* (Vol 19, pp. 28–39). London: Hogarth Press. (Original work published 1923).

Freud, S. (1975d). The dependent relationships of the ego. In J. Strachey (Ed. and Trans.), *The standard edition of the complete psychological works of Sigmund Freud* (Vol. 19, pp. 48–59). London: Hogarth Press. (Original work published 1923).

Gutheil T. G., & Gabbard G. O. (1993). The concept of boundaries in clinical practice: Theoretical risk-management. *American Journal of Psychiatry, 150*, 188–196. https://ajp. psychiatryonline.org/ (accessed on 4th August 2023).

Hartmann, E. (1991). *Boundaries in the mind: A new psychology of personality*. New York: Basic Books.

Hartmann, E. (1997). The concept of boundaries in counselling and psychotherapy. *British Journal of Guidance & Counselling, 25*(2), 147–162. Taylor & Francis Online. https:// doi.org/10.1080/03069889700760141.

Landreth, G. (1991). *Play therapy: The art of the relationship*. New York: Accelerated Development Inc. Taylor Francis Group.

Lavering, D. (2014). *The relationships between attachment style and boundary thickness.* (Dissertations & Theses). 245. http://aura.antioch.edu/etds/245

Lewin, R. A. (1994). Boundaries in clinical psychiatry. *American Journal of Psychiatry, 151*(2), 294.

Minuchin, S. (1974). *Families and family therapy*. Cambridge, MA: Harvard University Press.

O'Sullivan, L., & Ryan, V. (2009). Therapeutic limits from an attachment perspective. *Clinical Child Psychology and Psychiatry, 14*(2), 215–235. Sage.

Owen, I. (1997). Boundaries in the practice of humanistic counselling. *British Journal of Guidance and Counselling, 25*(2), 163–174.

Pinney, R. (1983). *Bobby: Breakthrough of an autistic child*. London: Harvill Press Ltd.

Rodgers, N. (2009). Therapeutic letters a challenge to conventional notions of boundary. *Journal of Family Nursing*. February, *15*(1), 50–64. © 2009 Sage Publications.

Rowan, J., & Jacobs, M. (2002). *The therapist's use of self*. Buckingham, UK: Open University Press.

Rumi. *A great wagon* (13th century).

Sandseter, E. B. H., & Kennair, L. E. O. (2011). Children's risky play from an evolutionary perspective: The anti-phobic effects of thrilling experiences. *Evolutionary Psychology, 9*, 257–284.

Winnicott, D. W. (1958). *Collected papers: Through paediatrics to psycho-analysis*. New York: Basic Books.

Woskett, V. (1999). *The therapeutic use of self: Counselling practice, research and supervision*. London: Routledge.

Postcards from the playroom

As I have mentioned, I worked for many years with a specialist therapy team providing support for children and young people with problematic and harmful sexual behaviour. As one might imagine, we worked with a range of challenging behaviours and associated sexual predilections, clinically termed paraphilia, which generally means atypical and often quite fetishistic recurrent sexual behaviours.

I recall working with an adolescent with learning disabilities who had a very particular and persistent sexual interest in feet. During one session, he wanted to play a game of hide and seek, not uncommon in play therapy, and he asked me to close my eyes. I told him that I did not feel comfortable closing my eyes but agreed to compromise by looking away for a few moments. Disconcerted by the rustling sounds, I turned around to find him in what looked like the act of masturbating into his shoe (thankfully not mine). I pondered for a moment upon the appropriate, empathic therapeutic reflection or how I might utilise Landreth's ACT model of limit-setting, but in the end just yelped out something like *Stop that . . . now!* It was not perhaps the most therapeutic response, but again, it was not something that came up in training, so to speak. Anyway, just be careful when you play hide and seek – you never quite know what you might find.

Chapter 9

Weather report

The climate emergency and child mental health

'I want you to panic. I want you to feel the fear I feel every day. And then I want you to act'. These were the words of environmental activist Greta Thunberg, speaking at the Davos World Economic Forum, in January 2019. Thunberg was 8 years old when she first became aware of the issue of climate change, and of the impact this was having upon her emotional well-being. She was 15 when she began her *school strike for climate* campaign, protesting outside the Swedish Parliament every Friday, a campaign that quickly picked up momentum around the world as more and more young people joined the school strikes. On the 1st March 2019, 150 students from the global coordination group of the youth-led climate strike movement, including Thunberg, issued an open letter in the *Guardian*.

> We, the young, are deeply concerned about our future. We are the voiceless future of humanity. We will no longer accept this injustice. We finally need to treat the climate crisis as a crisis. It is the biggest threat in human history and we will not accept the world's decision-makers' inaction that threatens our entire civilisation. Climate change is already happening. People did die, are dying and will die because of it, but we can and will stop this madness. United we will rise until we see climate justice. We demand the world's decision-makers take responsibility and solve this crisis. You have failed us in the past. If you continue failing us in the future, we, the young people, will make change happen by ourselves. The youth of this world has started to move and we will not rest again.
>
> (2019)

It is interesting that it took a child to bring the climate emergency to public attention; that it took thousands of school children from across the world to embed this message into our collective consciousness. Of course, whilst the climate crisis is affecting everyone right now, in the longer-term it is the younger generation who have the most to fear and the most to lose. Indeed, what is striking about Thunberg's opening quote to this chapter is firstly the sense of trauma it conveys – the panic and fear – and secondly, the sense of helplessness; that her very future is in the hands of others. This is the very essence of trauma; an experience of inescapable

DOI: 10.4324/9781003352563-9

fear and an inability to affect the outcome of your situation – a rising sense of feeling trapped, an acute emotional parallel to the rising level of heat trapped within our atmosphere.

Thunberg and the millions other young people across the globe are, both metaphorically and literally, the gaslit generation, subjected to the false reality of politicians, fiscal institutions and global corporations, who with one hand offer pledges of net zero emissions, reduced carbon footprints and the ending of deforestation, and with the other hand reel in the massive profits generated by their so-called climate solutions. Green gaslighting is an act of mass deception, a corporate sleight of hand, that both deceives and disempowers. Also striking about Thunberg's words is the sense of urgency they convey; an anxious plea to those with power and influence, as she desperately seeks to hand the responsibility back to where it belongs and lift the burden from her own young shoulders. And therein lies the existential paradox; that the future well-being of Thunberg and her generation depends upon the actions of others, who through inaction, incompetence, corruption or plain deceit, are also the greatest source of threat. It is a trauma dynamic that therapists are only all too familiar with.

The aim of this chapter is to look at the consequences of this felt burden and the impact of the climate emergency upon the emotional health and well-being of children and young people. Specifically, it will explore the implications for therapists, who (still reeling from the psychological consequences of the Covid-19 pandemic) may well find themselves in the front-line, facing the rising tide of a new public mental health challenge. I will seek to look at the therapeutic implications of both the impact of eco-anxiety, the chronic, enduring and cumulative sense of environmental, existential threat felt by many young people, and the more direct consequences of those who have been physically impacted by climate change i.e. those who have been displaced through fires, floods or storms.

I also need to declare my bias here; in that I am an active member of what can loosely be termed the 'environmental movement'. But this is not a debate about climate change per se; it is not even a debate about how and where we might position ourselves in relation to the climate change question. It is though, a debate about the unquestionable impact that the issue of climate change is having upon the mental health of children and young people, and how as therapists we can best support these young people.

Eco-anxiety

In 2022, the UK hit record high temperatures, peaking at just over 40 degrees. I remember standing in my garden, rendered motionless by the heat, the air thick like treacle and the neighbourhood eerily subdued, with even the birds stunned into a muted submission. I remember a pervasive sense of strangeness, a sense that the weather simply felt 'wrong'. On the radio, I listened to reports of firefighters battling hundreds of blazes around the country, people dying of heat exhaustion, people drowning whilst attempting to avoid heat exhaustion, planes grounded by melting runways and trains halted by buckling rails. Across Europe, a series of heatwaves contributed to the worst droughts for hundreds of years. Many countries across Europe, notably Spain, were ravaged by wildfires. In Pakistan, historic flooding affected the lives of more than 33 million people, and caused at least 1400 deaths. Sea surface temperatures across large areas of the North Atlantic were the warmest on record. Hurricanes, with rather friendly, incongruent names like Ian and Nicole, battered large areas of the Caribbean and the US. And as I write this now in the summer of 2023, as a new, unprecedented heatwave sweeps across southern Europe, the past tense has become redundant. This is now our present and future reality. It is a sobering thought that the process of writing this chapter cannot keep up with the pace of the current climate crisis engulfing our planet.

It is a reality that is played out through the media, a relentless cycling of news stories as the climate records tumble; highest temperatures, fiercest storms, worst floods, most deaths. Social media recycles these stories, moving the news from the global to the personal, an online wildfire that – as only social media can – amplifies and spins the messaging. And as is often the way, I find myself all too easily sucked into this news cycle, endlessly doomscrolling my way through the relentless reports, pictures and stories of our changing climate. I watch images of people clinging to the roof of their house hoping to get airlifted to safety, whole towns burned to the ground, children starving as they face another year of drought, bridges swept away by torrential floods and forlorn, stunted glaciers in melting retreat. It is an unhealthy diet in terms of self-care, and I wonder about its emotional impact.

As we know, anxiety will manifest itself in all manner of ways and there are various protective defence strategies that we can both consciously and unconsciously employ to defend, deny, avoid, displace, suppress, repress etc. I find it hard to know exactly what I feel in response to this media barrage; a cumulative sense of emotional numbing perhaps, detachment, resignation, worry, helplessness and at times frustration and anger. But underneath all these feelings there is I think an underlying anxiety, and whilst low-level anxiety in the face of the stark reality of climate change is a normal response, for some the experience of climate related eco-anxiety will have a serious, debilitating impact upon their lives, leading to significant emotional and psychological distress.

I am also aware that my response to the climate crisis will differ to others, and that the way people respond will be dependent upon a range of variable factors, for example age, knowledge, resilience, support networks, neuro-diversity, health and pre-existing anxiety related conditions. Some people then, maybe more predisposed to eco-anxiety than others, and researchers (Léger-Goodes, Malboeuf-Hurtubise et al., 2022) have suggested that the concept of eco-anxiety could be placed on something of a spectrum. On one end of this spectrum, our strong, emotional responses to the reporting of climate change might lead to action and mobilisation, enabling a sense of control and empowerment, for example changing our behaviours or getting directly involved in the environmental movement. At the other end of the spectrum, the experience of eco-anxiety might leave one feeling helpless and disempowered, with the overwhelming enormity of the issue creating a debilitating sense of paralysis. On a personal level, I find myself oscillating between these two points; sometimes mobilised and active in doing what I can to engage in the issue, at other times more a sense of defeated resignation. But I have choices and a sense of personal agency, which is not necessarily the same for all children and young people.

The term *eco-anxiety* is commonly used to describe what Pihkala (2018) defines as the 'emotional and mental states associated with heightened awareness of climate change and concurrent distress in the face of its threatening implications for the future' (2018: 53). Whilst not (yet) included in the DSM-5 (Diagnostic and Statistical Manual of Mental Disorders) it is a term that reflects the growing recognition of the links between climate change and mental health, what Clayton et al. (2017) describe as a 'chronic fear of environmental doom'. Like any mental health label, *eco-anxiety* can be a problematic term, potentially pathologising an emotional/psychological response to a very real threat, once again a rather gaslit dynamic, whilst also failing to capture the complex, wide-ranging constellation of emotional responses to this environmental threat, for example helplessness, powerlessness, guilt, anger, grief, loss and despair. Similarly, it is important that the labelling of 'eco-anxiety' does not privilege the problem/solution as being within the sole domain of an individual mental health context, negating the need for wider, systemic change (and to position the problem where it belongs). Others (Van Susteren, 2021; Kaplan, 2020) have interestingly used the term 'pre-traumatic stress disorder' to describe the traumatic anticipation of felt consequences before the event, including symptoms like 'flash-forwards' and fear induced dissociation, although I would suggest that the term 'pre-traumatic' is something of a misnomer; the trauma is present and real, here and now.

Alongside eco-anxiety, the term *solastalgia* is also increasingly being used within the lexicon of the climate crisis to describe the sense of 'distress or desolation caused by the gradual removal of solace from the present state of one's home environment' (Albrecht, 2011: 50). It is a poignant term, capturing the grief and existential distress caused by environmental change, a sense of homesickness without leaving home, a mourning for one's lost or changing homeland. This might be through drought or fire, the crisis driven events that leave a permanent, incremental change upon the landscape, but solastalgia is a term that perhaps applies most aptly to those indigenous populations who live in particularly fragile environments where the impact of climate change is both increasingly rapid and which has a direct impact upon the lives (and livelihoods) of the inhabitants. For example, in the Artic, the Inuit traditions of hunting, fishing and harvesting, those generational patterns of living alongside their environment, are being disrupted as climate change disturbs seasonal cycles and access to land and water. Solastalgia is also a poignant term in relation to mental health, invoking not the anxiety of future threat, but rather the aching, real-time melancholy of everyday loss.

I recall being in New Zealand, just weeks before Covid-19 closed the world down. We were visiting Mount Aoraki/Cook and had hiked up the Hooker Valley Track that leads to the ever-retreating head of the Hooker Glacier. We noticed that the streaks of ice and snow lying in the shadowed crevices of the mountain-side were tinged a dirty brown, a consequence of the ferocious bush fires that at the same time were sweeping across areas of South Eastern Australia, on the other side of the Tasman Sea. In years to come there will be a brown timeline in the ice, a geological record of the event. At the head of the trail, small icebergs floated eerily in the brown waters of Hooker Lake, having broken off from the main glacier. It was a stunning sight, but also sad. Even as we stood looking across the lake to the glacier, there were occasional, startling booms, like the sound of distant cannon fire, which echoed across the valley and we saw large chunks of ice break off and slip almost shamefully into the brown waters of the lake. Climate change was happening right there and then, in front of our very eyes. Talking later to a member of the team at the Mount Aoraki Information Centre, we were told that they see climate related change happening on a daily basis. But what struck me most was the tragic synchronicity that saw one catastrophic climate change event captured in another, the burning fires and the melting ice, a dramatic example of the interconnectedness of the climate crisis and the systemic impact this change is having upon the planet. Although both beautiful and awe inspiring, our hike to the Hooker Glacier was also a profoundly sad moment that brought home the full meaning and context of solastalgia.

The emotional impact of the climate crisis on children and young people

In one of the largest studies to date (Hickman, Marks, Pihkala et al., 2021), 10,000 children and young people across ten countries were asked about their emotional response to climate change. The findings of this survey provided a striking picture, with 59% of respondents stating that they felt 'worried' or 'extremely worried' about climate change. Furthermore, over 60% of respondents reported feeling afraid, sad and/or anxious, and at least 50% reported feeling angry, powerless, helpless and/or guilty. Perhaps surprisingly, 40% of respondents stated that their concerns around the climate emergency have led them to think twice about having children.

A key theme that emerged from this study was that of generational betrayal, leading the authors to argue that the failure of governments to adequately address, tackle or even acknowledge the urgency of climate change is a key contributory factor to the experience of climate related psychological distress. This sense of betrayal can only compound feelings of helplessness and abandonment and from a psychotherapy perspective the analogy once again is that of a failure to protect; the traumatised child dependent upon the abusive, neglectful parent. Thunberg's emotional plea is to *feel the fear* – a call not to arms but to empathy and compassion, precious qualities that seem in short supply within the climate debate.

It may not be a safeguarding issue, as we usually understand the term, but it is arguably a social justice/human rights issue, an act of moral injury. Interestingly, within this context there is growing phenomena of climate criminology (White, 2015) in which children and young people are beginning to seek recourse through the courts, to legally challenge the authorities by whom they feel so betrayed. This may be a route of limited success, but perhaps this is more about a desire for empowerment, an attempt by young people to have their fear and distress legitimised in the face of government inaction. Certainly, the feelings of young people who responded to the aforementioned survey were validated by the report's authors, who acknowledged feeling 'disturbed' by the scale of the emotional impact that climate change is having upon young people around the world. As they state,

> we wish that these results had not been quite so devastating. The global scale of this study is sufficient to warrant a warning to governments and adults around the world, and it underscores an urgent need for greater responsiveness to children and young people's concerns, more in-depth research, and immediate action on climate change.
>
> (2021: 872)

The relationship between climate change and mental health (Lawrance et al., 2022) is a deeply complex, multi-systemic picture; the dynamic interaction between a range of socio/economic/political factors may lead individuals, or indeed communities, to be more vulnerable to the psychological impact of the climate emergency. Like Covid-19, climate change starkly exposes those societal, intersectional fault lines that invariably, inevitably, lead some people or communities to be more vulnerable than others. In a move to capture and communicate this level of complexity, Imperial College researchers Lawrance et al. (2022) developed a systemic framework/model (2022: 448) to highlight the 'multiple interacting layers of influence' (2022: 444) that might impact upon an individual's mental health. As illustrated within this model, and discussed elsewhere in this book, the dynamics of power, privilege and oppression are an ever-present part of this picture, and as the preceding authors note, the western legacies of 'colonialism and conflict' (2022: 447) have their own story to tell when it comes to the politics of climate change. Those more economically disadvantaged communities, with the allied factors of poor housing, health outcomes, air quality, access to greenspace etc will be disproportionately affected and as the authors suggest 'for communities already facing complex disadvantage, climate change can act as a risk multiplier and exacerbates existing inequalities and vulnerabilities, including in mental health' (2022: 447).

As Berry et al. (2018) have suggested, the mental health impact of climate change can be thought about in terms of three distinct categories; direct, indirect and vicarious. Direct impact includes exposure to extreme weather events such as floods, fires, storms etc, all of which will clearly have both an immediate and a post-traumatic mental health impact. The more indirect mental health impacts include those of displacement, climate migration, food and water shortages and longer-term issues of economy, housing and education. These are all factors that will have a significant impact upon children's mental health and well-being, including anxiety, developmental trauma, depression and the multiple consequences of familial stress.

But beyond these direct and indirect consequences are the more displaced, vicarious effects of climate change, for example through children's exposure to television, news, social media, parental anxiety and their growing educational awareness of climate related issues. Although less researched, there is growing evidence to suggest that this kind of exposure to the effects of climate change can lead to vicarious eco-anxiety, for example feelings of being overwhelmed, fearfulness, obsessive thinking, panic attacks and sleep disturbance. For therapists, it is this more indirect and vicarious emotional impact of the climate crisis that they are likely to see in their clinics, as children struggle to process and make sense of the developing climate story.

As suggested by Vergunst and Berry (2021), establishing a causal pathway from climate change related exposure to children's mental health is complex and challenging. Clearly, exposure to the direct impact of extreme weather events, as highlighted earlier, will have an immediate impact upon children's mental health as well as their physical safety; causality in this context can be easily observed and understood. But the causal effects upon children of the more indirect, longer-term and vicarious exposure to climate related events, for example through television, school, peers, parents etc is harder to evidence, being more displaced, variable and diffuse. Similarly, distinguishing what we might think of as normal worry from more acute, clinical anxiety is challenging and as Hayes et al. (2018) suggested, there is a risk of pathologising emotional responses to other adverse life events and misattributing these to the climate crisis, or alternatively failing to recognise how the exposure to the climate crisis may be affecting a child's mental well-being. Indeed as we know as therapists, children themselves often do not know what it is that might be contributing or causing their experience of anxiety, or do not have the capacity to verbally articulate their worries.

So, whilst there is little literature or clinical research evidencing children's experiences of eco-anxiety, as with the 2001 Twin Towers terrorist attack, the 2004 tsunami and more recently, Covid-19 and the war in Ukraine, the climate crisis seeps into children's growing awareness, both conscious and unconscious, with related themes and images beginning to appear in their play. Anecdotally, as I talk with other colleagues and professionals within the therapeutic community, there is an emerging picture of children being emotionally affected by the climate crisis and consequently it is important that we think about how children, young people and their families can best be supported.

Implications for therapy: supporting children with eco-anxiety

Child centred play therapy

As we know, child centred play therapy (Landreth, 1991; Axline, 1984) is a developmentally appropriate and well-evidenced (Bratton et al., 2005) therapeutic approach for supporting younger children. That said, there will be developmental differences in the way that children and young people are emotionally impacted by the climate crisis. Whilst middle childhood is an exciting period of active cognitive, social and emotional development, it is also a period of developmental vulnerability as children become more emotionally independent and susceptible to influence from peers, teachers, the internet and social media. Children are acutely aware of parental stress, and climate anxiety experienced by parents is likely to be felt by children, albeit in a more generalised and non-specific manner. Younger children are less able to cognitively process and contextualise the political/social/economic factors associated with climate change, but may well communicate their worries in non-verbal and less conscious ways, for example oppositional or obsessive behaviours, over-compliance, emotional withdrawal or sleeping and eating difficulties. In my experience, children generally know more than their parents think they know, but in the absence of age-appropriate explanation and information this unprocessed awareness is likely to translate into generalised and displaced anxiety related behaviours.

Within the preceding context, it is often hard to know the underlying reason that a child might present with anxiety. There are many other potential societal stressors alongside the current climate crisis, for example the continuing legacy of Covid, war in Ukraine, the cost-of-living crisis and, of course, the specific individual and familial factors that may be impacting upon a child's life. Indeed, it may well be a combination of several of these factors. But given the opportunity for creative play within a safe, contained environment and supportive relationship, children can find ways to express and explore what they need to.

Recently, I worked with a young boy who had been referred for play therapy due to his experience of generalised anxiety, which was having a detrimental impact upon both his life and that of the family. During the sessions, the boy spoke of his more specific fear of being murdered in the night by a stranger. Being quite a literal child, I took quite a cognitive approach and suggested that his parents share what the statistics show about the actual numbers of children who get murdered by strangers in their own home – a kind of reality testing of the fact against the fantasy. It also became apparent that from his bedroom he could hear his parents watching the news on television, perhaps unhelpful for a child prone to anxiety.

But I also invited him to use the sandtray to show me what this fear might look like and he created a frightening world of fearsome, giant spiders, buried monsters and scary creatures. In the middle of this world was an oasis of water, plants and precious stones. It was a symbolic expression of his internal world, his fears and fantasies, and whilst not specifically about climate change, I was struck by the metaphor. Is it not what we all fear on some deep, primal level? The fear of being killed in the night? The safe, sanctuary of home being threatened by some unknown, faceless intruder? The outside, pressing in? Climate change represents an existential threat, one of many, and while it is hard to know what lies beneath children's experiences of non-specific, generalised anxiety, it is important that we are alert to the possible symbolism within their play; clues perhaps to their internal world.

Hickman (2020) describes interviewing a 10-year-old boy about his feelings in relation to climate change. The boy's father was rather dismissive, explaining that his son probably did not even know what climate change was. But much to the father's surprise, his son then proceeded to describe climate change as a gigantic crocodile, the size of a continent –

> and it was crawling over the face of the earth, crawling out of the shadows. It had to keep eating and eating, it would never stop, but would never have eaten enough. And it was rotting from the inside out, scales were falling away as it crawled forwards, rotting and eating. And you could smell its dying flesh as it still ate and ate and ate.
>
> (2020: 421)

Hickman poignantly describes the father's growing shock as his son painted a metaphorical but graphic picture of the 'interrelationship between climate change, consumption, economic growth, polluting destructive industrial practices, the juxtaposition of consumption and destruction, death and extinction. All themes very relevant to climate change' (2020: 421).

They are themes that I recognise from many of the anxious children that I have worked with, particularly that of over-consumption; the insatiable monster devouring more and more of the world around it. As Carbis (2022) states, the way in which adults approach the issue of climate change with their children will vary greatly, depending upon a range of variable factors, for example their own awareness and understanding of the issue, their beliefs, values and attitudes and their confidence in finding helpful and appropriate ways to talk to their children. But these conversations are important, just as it is that children can be supported in finding creative, playful and safe ways to tell their stories. Play therapy can play an important role in this process and as Carbis states, 'play therapists have a responsibility to educate themselves about climate change and the impact it is having on children's mental health and wellbeing' (2022: 72).

Nature-based play therapy

Climate change occurs within a complex, eco-systemic context. It is a crisis literally rooted in the natural world and its response to the threat posed by human activity. The balance of our natural world, the ecology of our planet, is delicately poised and whilst nature will often find its way, it could be suggested that we, the human component of this delicate connected system, are beginning to lose ours. And as an (albeit human-engineered) crisis of the natural world, an appropriate and congruent therapeutic approach to supporting children experiencing eco-anxiety is through ecology itself. Children's understanding and experience of environmental change is largely informed by the stark, media driven imagery of storms, floods and fires. In this sense, the environment becomes something dangerous and fearful, and so the notion of the natural environment as a source of emotional sustenance and nurture is an important counterpoint to this imagery. In this sense, nature can be a great healer.

Fearn (2022) writes about the role of nature as a therapeutic ally for the play therapist. As Fearn states, 'immersive play experiences in the natural environment promote a child's growth, development and healing, and evoke the possibilities, wonder and limits of being a human being' (2022: 1). Life is interconnected; a rich, complex, magical entanglement, no better symbolised than by the interwoven, mycelium fungal threads that taken together make up the mycorrhizal network of our woodlands and forests; connecting, distributing and regulating the transfer of water, nitrogen, carbon and other valuable nutrients and minerals. These complex organic networks of roots, threads and micro-filaments are not unlike the interconnected neural pathways of the human brain/body system; the synapses and nodes, the neuro-transmitters and chemical messengers, those delicate mechanisms that regulate our neurobiology – or perhaps in this context, our neuroecology. The complex neuroendocrine pathways of the HPA (hypothalamic-pituitary-adrenal) axis that functions to maintain our sense of homeostasis and physiological equilibrium is in many ways analogous to nature's regulating mycorrhizal network and, as is ever the way, perhaps nature can help us find a way forward.

As has been explored elsewhere in this book, we are living in a world that is seemingly becoming increasingly disconnected and polarised, more either/or than both/and. There is no more stark and serious illustration of this than the present climate emergency; a crisis that demands social cooperation and collaboration but is instead met with political short-term isolationism and protectionism. But as nature shows us, life is deeply interconnected and mutually interdependent. As Fearn suggests,

> all species within a natural community cooperate with each other. Survival depends on being entangled with other species, belonging in relationship to each other and with those yet to be born, including all species who directly or indirectly live off and with the land, the air and the water that flows through it.
>
> (2022: 2)

Children too can become disconnected from the natural world around them, perhaps compounding feelings of eco-anxiety, and one way to mitigate the impact of this anxiety is to facilitate their positive relationship with their environment and help them feel a part of this natural community, itself a wonderful therapist. As I discuss in Chapter 1 of this book, we can become attached to nature and place, as we can to people, and just as we know that play is intrinsically healing, so it is with nature, a fact increasingly borne out through research (Engemann et al., 2019; Bratman et al, 2019; Reyes-Riveros et al., 2021).

Nature informed play therapists who, as Fearn so eloquently describes, engage with nature as a therapeutic ally in their work with troubled children, will bear testimony to the restorative and reparative qualities of the natural world. Carbis (2022) writes of the benefits of nature-based climate change therapeutic groups, emphasising how community orientated action can be effective in mitigating the anxiety caused by the climate crisis. Whilst there is a growing body of research evidencing the benefits of nature-based, outdoor play, as Carbis (2022) has highlighted, some critics might argue that if children spend time appreciating the therapeutic value of nature, their feelings of anxiety and loss might be exacerbated by becoming closer to the very nature they fear losing. Carbis counters that this appears to be a minority response, the hope being that the therapeutic benefits of being in nature will encourage children and young people into action, itself an emotionally protective factor. As Carbis states, the 'use of nature therapeutically is not only a medium that children who have concerns about the climate crisis will likely feel comfortable with and benefit from, but this involvement with nature may also inspire more pro-environmental behaviour' (2022: 70).

Nature-based play can help children to become attuned to their natural environment; to understand the interconnectedness of natural cycles and systems and develop a curiosity about the world around them. Nature is also a wonderful emotional regulator; be it the sensation of soft grass under one's feet, the earthy smell of moss, the ephemeral flash of a butterfly's wing or passing companionship of a curious robin. Herein lies the essence of neuroecology, the active, mutual, healing relationship between the two systems, mycorrhizal and neural, that can regulate affect and mitigate the impact of anxiety and emotional distress. In turn, this may help children develop a greater awareness of our relationship to the natural world and the finely tuned balance of the ecosystem. Anxiety, as we know, often occupies the space between knowledge and fantasy – the fear of the unknown. Climate change is a part of the delicate pattern of life, and if children can become more aware and informed of the relationship between humans, climate and the world that we share, then this might help take away some of the fear around environmental change.

The role of carers and families

Children's exposure to and awareness of the climate crisis is mainly through their parents, school and news/social media. Peer influence is likely to be less with younger children but will significantly increase as they get older. Parents' values, beliefs, attitudes and knowledge around climate change is likely to be reflected in their children, and as children are generally highly attuned to their parents' emotional states, any anxiety around climate change is likely to be picked up. Conversely, there is also research (Lawson et al., 2019) suggesting that children's eco-anxiety can contribute to their parent's level of environmental concern, so there is a danger that families can become stuck within a pattern of negative rein-forcement. A study by Léger-Goodes et al. (2022) suggested that whilst parents consider themselves both models and educators in relation to climate change, this is done more through pro-environmental behaviours such as recycling rather than teaching their children coping strategies or sharing their thoughts and feelings re climate change. The suggestion within this study is that the potential shame, guilt or anxiety experienced by parents may lead them to avoid the subject with their children.

The clinical, practice implication of this potential pattern of mutual avoidance is the importance of including parents and carers in the therapeutic process and to support them in being able to both listen to their children and engage them in hon-est discussions about the climate crisis. As said, there is potential for a collusive, unspoken avoidance of the issue, perhaps as a result of uncertainty or incongruent values, attitudes and beliefs and in this sense, it is also important for us as thera-pists to ensure that we are as informed as possible and aware of our own potential blind-spots, unconscious bias and implicit assumptions. Equally, it is important that therapists support parents in finding ways to engage their children in positive, empowering and mobilising activities as a way of increasing a sense of personal agency and reducing climate related anxiety.

The climate crisis is systemic, just as is therapy, and as influential advocates for the children we work with, it is important that we support the networks around chil-dren to find connected, collective and community-based ways in which to enrich, nourish and nurture their lives as a counterpoint to the debilitating and paralysing impact of climate anxiety. To draw from the aforementioned nature-based analogy, it is an opportunity to mobilise the protective, social mycorrhizal eco-system that can provide such an important network for children and families. Collective action brings hope and hope brings the possibility of change.

Finding a way forward: the importance of hope

'To live without hope is to cease to live.'

(Fyodor Dostoevsky)

As I know only too well myself, it can be hard to hold on to a position of hope and optimism when faced with what feels like the increasingly desperate reality of climate change. The language and vocabulary of climate change is littered with doom-laden nouns like *emergency*, *crisis* and *disaster*, words that rise like forbid-ding, impassable mountains in the treacherous, insurmountable lexicon of the cli-mate landscape. It can be hard to navigate a way through this terrain, particularly when weighed down by anxiety and the sense that there is little that one can do to affect change.

Research (Strife, 2012) found that 82% of children expressed fear, sadness and anger when talking about environmental issues, with the majority of the children also sharing apocalyptic and pessimistic feelings about the future state of the planet. Further research (Kelsey & Armstrong, 2012) has suggested that feelings of climate related pessimism develop in late childhood and increase into the later years of adolescence. But within this somewhat bleak picture it is also important to hold onto the potential role of hope as a protective factor and an important part of the supportive framework that can strengthen children's well-being and enable them to effectively engage with the issue of climate change. The question here is how we, whether in the position of therapist, parent or educator, can help children and young people to develop a more positive and empowered narrative around the climate crisis, and I would suggest that a critical part of this narrative is the presence of hope.

Hope has been defined as 'the perceived capability to derive pathways to desired goals, and motivate oneself via agency thinking to use those pathways' (Snyder, 2002: 249). This definition emphasises three specific elements: *goals, pathways* and *agency*, elements further characterised by Olsson (2020) as 'knowledge, confidence and the will to act'. Action then, is intrinsic to hope and this is particularly relevant to the climate crisis, the vernacular of which all too easily tips into a narrative of despair and despondency. As Frumkin (2022) notes, these doom-laden narratives can have a significant impact on young people's responses to the climate crisis, not just in terms of emotion, but also in relation to their future life choices, for example forgoing higher education in the belief that it is pointless, or choosing not to have children. In a survey of child and adolescent psychiatrists (Royal College of Psychiatrists 2020) in England, over 50% reported treating children and young people experiencing climate change related distress, with many citing feelings of hopelessness. It is then, it could be argued, incumbent upon us as therapists and mental health professionals to counter these climate narratives of hopelessness and as Frumkin argues, there are at least three compelling, evidence-based reasons to do so, namely that 'hopeful people feel better than hopeless people', 'hope leads to action' and 'hope is empirically justified' (2022: 3).

Hope sustains agency and vice versa, creating a virtuous circle that can regulate worry and climate-based anxiety. As Buchanan et al. (2021) suggest in their paper outlining a pedagogy of hope, the 'stronger the sense of hope in the face of climate change among young people, the more likely the related positive outcomes because of their proactive engagement' (2021: 3). A constructive sense of hope is more likely to lead to positive, pro-environmental behaviours, whether in the form of political engagement and activism or the making of those everyday lifestyle choices that enable people to feel that they can make a positive difference. In essence, it is about meaningful activity and the development of coping strategies that can foster a greater sense of emotional resilience and self-efficacy. Linked to this is the importance of mutual collaboration, to feel part of a community of others joined in a common aim.

Anxiety can be lonely and isolating, creating a sense of helplessness and emotional dislocation and so an experience of connection and collaboration, driven by a collective sense of hope, can be very powerful. I have felt for myself the deeply restorative experience of joining thousands of others, acting together towards a shared goal of environmental justice. Indeed, it is hope made tangible; an embodied, mutual, expression of the desire for change, a collective will to act, that can combat the anxiety around the climate crisis, the scope and enormity of which can often feel all too overwhelming. It has also been very moving to witness young children's participation in these forms of collective action, that they also can experience this power of community. Recently, I took part in an environmental march and walking close by were a couple with their two young children. Every now and again the crowd would break out into a call and response chant. *What do we want? Climate justice. When do we want it? Now.* The children joined in, at times leading the chant, and whilst I am aware of the need to be mindful that involving children in such activities does not compound any potential anxiety they may be experiencing, as I watched these children, smiling, eager and energised, and saw the strength of affirmation they received from the crowd and the demonstrable love and support of their parents, I felt I was witnessing the very special power of the collective spirit.

Kelsey (2016) talks about the power of climate related emotional contagion; hope is infectious, as is despair, and within this context she asks the key question; 'how do we propagate hope when we ourselves are inundated by doom and gloom?' (2016: 24). As therapists, we know all too well about the impact of emotional contagion; the impact of vicarious trauma and the creeping stealth of the unconscious process. The climate crisis is also traumatic; listen again to Thunberg's words that open this chapter. Environmental news is invariably reported as 'bad news' and is understandably framed within the pervasive but compelling story arc of the 'disaster narrative'. But unlike the disaster movies of the big screen, there is no heroic saviour or magic bullet, or comfort-blanket final scene that sees the young child pulled out of a burning building at the last moment and safely reunited with their family. We do not know how this story ends, or the problem is that perhaps we do, and within this lived experience it is increasingly hard to hold on to a sense of optimism. Again, as therapists, we know about the importance of hope in our work, but as Kelsey highlights, the language of hope is conspicuously absent from environmental discourse, a feature that can only both contribute to and compound the experience of climate related anxiety.

So, perhaps then as therapists we have an important role and responsibility in facilitating hopefulness in the children and young people who we are working with so that we do not, as Kelsey puts it, inadvertently perpetuate a legacy of fear. But importantly, this is also not about creating 'false hope' and as Kelsey states, 'hope in this context is not conceptualized in terms of the promise of a better future; it is grounded in a sense of a meaningful present' (2016: 28). I have worked with many children who have had extreme experiences of abuse, trauma and neglect. My work has not been able to take way those experiences of abuse; they are a fact, a given, that cannot be undone. But the process of therapy can enable children to live a meaningful life alongside these experiences, so that they can experience healthy, sustaining relationships and regain a sense of control, albeit within a context of troubled pasts and often uncertain futures. Similarly (although not a comparison) we cannot take away the reality of climate change, but we can enable young people to process this reality and help them and their families negotiate their way through this uncertain terrain, to help them find personally meaningful coping strategies and ultimately, maintain a sense of hope and agency.

Hope then, is an important protective factor that can counteract the all too pervasive and negative narratives that permeate the climate change debate. As therapists, this is important for us to consider, in the context of the children, young people and families that we work with. The challenge lies in how we can both acknowledge the reality of the threat that the climate crisis presents whilst also nurturing and sustaining hope, in the midst of this crisis, whilst also having to hold onto hope ourselves. To this end, Frumkin (2022: 4) offers some strategies, or perhaps guiding principles, to health professionals as a way of legitimately propagating hope within our clinical practice:

1. *Tell the truth*

'With respect to climate change, two linked truths must be told: we confront a crisis; and there is much we can do. In clinical settings, patients want a balance between honesty and hope, a good model for truth-telling regarding climate change' (2022: 4).

2. *Acknowledge grief*

A beginning point for any therapeutic work around climate anxiety is the acknowledgement of grief and loss, not so much for the past or present, but for a future bereft of promise and potential – 'acknowledging the pain brings a sense of relief, hope, and increased determination and capacity to act' (2022: 4).

3. *Envision success*

Action and agency are intrinsic to hope. If children and young people can visualise the potential for positive change the more likely this can be translated into action and combat feelings of helplessness.

4. *Identify pathways to success*

Pathway thinking is a key element of hope and is part of identifying routes to achieve a desired goal. Within a therapeutic context this might be about exploring realistic and achievable ways to affect change.

5. *Empower people to act*

A part of the therapist role is to enable clients to consider the choices they have as a way of regaining a sense of control. On a personal level this might include pro-environmental behavioural changes and lifestyle choices and on a broader level, the advocating of systemic change.

6. *Cultivate solidarity*

Connection, collaboration and the sharing of mutually held goals can promote health and well-being and reduce feelings of anxiety. The experience of collective hope can be a powerful motivating factor.

7. *Make room for joy*

Happiness is synonymous with hopefulness and whilst climate change is a serious business it is also important to find ways to be playful and joyful. As the climate scientist Kim Nicholas (2020) says of climate action, it does not all have to be about sacrifice, suffering and despair; it can also be fun – 'there is so much joy in figuring out what really matters to you, living in line with those values and being part of a community of people who support each other' (2020). Personally, I have been struck by the playfulness, humour and creativity within the environmental movement and the sense that there is room for comfort, joy and celebration in people coming together in the spirit of shared, collective endeavour.

Therapist responsibility: a moral imperative?

It is important then for us as therapists to proactively engage in hope-orientated practice and support our clients in finding positive ways to challenge the often very pervasive narratives of 'doom and gloom' within the climate change story. This, as I know only all too well myself, is not always easy, but then without hope, what else is there? In the face of the growing climate crisis, it can be hard to hold onto a hopeful future, the danger being that we are all collectively dragged into the defeatist short-termism so beloved by our political elite. But as therapists we also know that the future is also informed by the past. Like the concept of cathedral thinking, even if we do not yet know how or when the roof is going to be built, we can still work towards the laying of a solid foundation, brick by brick, for the benefit of future generations.

But the challenge for us as therapists is how we might integrate these principles into our work whilst maintaining the core conditions that underpin our clinical practice. The case for authenticity and congruence seems clear, but where or how do we position ourselves in terms of judgement and neutrality? If, as suggested earlier, the climate crisis is also an issue of social justice and thereby represents a case of moral injury, what is our moral imperative as therapists?

I would suggest that the first step towards answering this question lies in the reflection upon our own values and attitudes in relation to the question of climate change; to know how to position ourselves we need to know what our position is. To be congruent requires personal clarity. In this sense, there is an ethical obligation to acknowledge our own thoughts, feelings and experiences around the climate crisis and to bring this into our conscious awareness when working with clients, whilst also being mindful of the unconscious processes, the patterns of transference and countertransference or unconscious bias that might impact, inform or influence the therapeutic relationship.

The climate crisis is also an existential crisis, raising powerful feelings around the meaning and significance of our lives and those of our future generations. It is a crisis that confronts us with the notion of a finite future and as Pihkala (2018) suggests, the association between climate change and mortality can generate powerful and unhelpful psychological defences, on both a conscious and unconscious level. Indeed, one could consider climate change denial as a psychological defence mechanism or coping strategy, the existential threat of the alternative being simply too much to bear. So, one of the tasks of therapy might be to find ways to explore those hidden feelings of fear and despair that might lie behind what Pihkala describes as the 'mask of apathy' (2018: 563). Finding and engaging with the power of hope might be the beginning part of this process.

Of course, we might also be in denial ourselves; we would be mistaken in believing that this lies within the sole domain of our clients. As therapists, we are also susceptible to the same existential fears and anxieties engendered by the climate crisis and the ongoing conflict between feelings of paralysis and mobilisation can affect our capacity to respond, react and 'step up' to the challenge. There is a difference between 'knowing' and 'doing'. We need to be mindful of our own process and how, where and why we might theoretically position ourselves re the question of climate change. We are facilitators and advocates, not activists, but that said, to be truly congruent means being open about our own internal process and the moral and ethical values that we hold dear to us within the context of our work. If we consider the climate crisis to be a social justice issue, then we have a just as great moral and ethical obligation to address, explore and potentially challenge this issue as we would with the power dynamics of oppression and discrimination.

My personal view is that we do, as therapists, have both a (personally) moral and (professionally) ethical obligation to address the issue of climate change within our work and to support those children, young people and families struggling with feelings around climate anxiety. Interestingly, some small-scale qualitative research around therapists' experience of climate change (Silva & Coburn, 2021) found that whilst therapists believed that there is an ethical obligation to address issues around climate anxiety (their own and their clients) within their practice, it is also an issue imbued with a complex range of conflictual feelings around therapist identity and parallel process – the 'experience of being unsettled and frustrated by their own sense of being complicit in the predicament of the climate crisis and its making' (2021: 424). Therein lies the clinical paradox; the internal conflictual and confusing feelings of being simultaneously both part of the problem and part of the solution. As the study states,

> each participant held the uncomfortable duality of an awareness of the anthropogenic nature of climate change and having good intentions on the one hand, and their own perceived but often unavoidable contribution to the problem in going about their day-to-day lives.

(202: 424)

The aforementioned study also highlights the urgent need for leadership, guidance and clinical governance from our professional bodies and training institutions to support therapists working within the growing and ever complex reality of the climate emergency. I have been struck personally by the seeming reluctance of professional bodies, including my own, to address this issue and rather than individual therapists having to grapple with the ethical dilemmas raised by the climate crises, it would surely be better for guidance to be integrated into our ethical frameworks for good practice, and this raises the question of organisational denial or at best, the absence of urgency. The climate crisis is a systemic crisis that demands systemic solutions, but we can be sure that time is not on our side. Perhaps we need to listen a little harder to the words of Greta Thunberg; that we need to panic, feel the fear . . . and act.

References

Albrecht, G. (2011). Chronic environmental change: Emerging 'psychoterratic' syndromes. In I. Weissbecker (Ed.), *Climate change and human well-being: Global challenges and opportunities* (pp. 43–56). New York: Springer.

Axline, V. M. (1984). *Play therapy*. London: Churchill Livingstone.

Berry, H., Waite, T. D., Dear, K. B. G., Capon, A. G., & Murray, V. (2018). The case for systems thinking about climate change and mental health. *Nature Climate Change, 8,* 282–290.

Bratman, G. et al. (2019). Nature and mental health: An ecosystem service perspective. *Science Advances, 5*(7).

Bratton, S. C., Ray, D., Rhine, T., & Jones, L. (2005). The efficacy of play therapy with children: A meta-analytic review of treatment outcomes. *Professional Psychology: Research and Practice, 36*(4), 376–390. https://doi.org/10.1037/0735-7028.36.4.376.

Buchanan, J., Pressick-Kilborn, K., & Fergusson, J. (2021). Naturally enough? Children, climate anxiety and the importance of hope. *Social Educator, 39*(3), 17–31.

Carbis, C. (2022). Play therapists response to the climate crisis. *British Journal of Play Therapy, 16,* 64–77. BAPT Publications.

Clayton, S., Manning, C. M., Krygsman, K., & Speiser, M. (2017). *Mental health and our changing climate: Impacts, implications, and guidance.* American Psychological Association, and ecoAmerica: Washington, DC. www.apa.org/news/press/releases/2017/03/mental-health-climate.pdf (accessed on 25th July 2023).

Engemann, K., Pederson, C. B., Arge, L., & Svenning, J. C. (2019). Residential green space in childhood is associated with lower risk of psychiatric disorders from adolescence into adulthood. *PNAS, 116*(11).

Fearn, M. (2022). Nature-based play therapy interventions in the digital age. In I. Cassina, C. Mochi, & K. Stagnitti (Eds.), *Play therapy and expressive arts in a complex and dynamic world: Opportunities and challenges inside and outside the playroom.* Abingdon, UK: Routledge.

Frumkin, H. (2022). Hope, health, and the climate crisis. *The Journal of Climate Change and Health, 5.* Elsevier.

Guardian (2019). *Climate crisis and a betrayed generation.* www.theguardian.com/environment/2019/mar/01/youth-climate-change-strikers-open-letter-to-world-leaders (accessed on 15th August 2023).

Hayes, K., Blashki, G., Wiseman, J., Burke, S., & Reifels, L. (2018). Climate change and mental health: Risks, impacts and priority actions. *International Journal of Mental Health Systems, 12,* 1–12.

Hickman, C. (2020). We need to (find a way) to talk about eco-anxiety. *Journal of Social Work Practice, 34*(4), 411–424.

Hickman, C., Marks, E., Pihkala, P., Clayton, S., Lewandowski, R. E., Mayall, E. E. et al. (2021). Climate anxiety in children and young people and their beliefs about government responses to climate change: A global survey. *Lancet Planet Health, 5*(12), e863–e873. https://doi.org/10.1016/S2542-5196(21)00278-3.

Kaplan, E. A. (2020). Is climate-related pre-traumatic stress syndrome a real condition? *American Imago, 77,* 81–104. https://doi.org/10.1353/aim.2020.0004.

Kelsey, E. (2016). Propagating collective hope in the midst of environmental doom and gloom. *The Canadian Journal of Environmental Education, 21.* Canada: Royal Roads University.

Kelsey, E., & Armstrong, C. (2012). Finding hope in a world of environmental catastrophe. In A. Wals & P. Corcoran (Eds.), *Learning for sustainability in times of accelerating change* (pp. 187–200). Wageningen, Netherlands: Wageningen Academic Publishers.

Landreth, G. (1991). *Play therapy: The art of the relationship.* New York: Accelerated Development Inc. Taylor Francis Group.

Lawrance, E., Thompson, R., Newberry Le Vay, J., Page, L., & Jennings, N. (2022). The impact of climate change on mental health and emotional wellbeing: A narrative review of current evidence, and its implications. *International Review of Psychiatry, 34*(5), 443–498. https://doi.org/10.1080/09540261.2022.2128725.

Lawson, D. F., Stevenson, K. T., Nils, P. M., Carrier, S. J., Renee, L. S., & Erin, S. (2019). Children can foster climate change concern among their parents. *Nature Climate Change, 9,* 458–462. https://doi.org/10.1038/s41558-019-0463-3.

Léger-Goodes, T., Malboeuf-Hurtubise, C., Mastine, T., Généreux, M., Paradis, P. O., & Chantal Camden, C. (2022). Eco-anxiety in children: A scoping review of the mental health impacts of the awareness of climate change. *Frontiers of Psychology.* 25 July. *Sec Environmental Psychology, 13.*

Nicholas, K. (2020). *We can all find purpose – And even joy – In responding to the climate crisis.* Transform21. Paris: International Science Council. https://council.science/current/blog/kim-nicholas-climate-crisis-interview/ (accessed on 25th July 2023).

Olsson, D. (2020). Self-perceived action competence for sustainability: The theoretical grounding and empirical validation of a novel research instrument. *Environmental Education Research, 26*(1), 1–19.

Pihkala, P. (2018). Eco-anxiety, tragedy, and hope: Psychological and spiritual dimensions of climate change. *Zygon, 53,* 545–569.

Reyes-Riveros, R. et al. (2021). Linking public urban green spaces and human well-being: A systematic review. *Urban Forestry and Greening, 61.* Elsevier.

Royal College of Psychiatrists (2020). *The climate crisis is taking a toll on the mental health of children and young people.* London. https://www.rcpsych.ac.uk/news-and-features/latest-news/detail/2020/11/20/the-climate-crisis-is-taking-a-toll-on-the-mental-health-of-children-and-young-people (accessed 25th July 2023).

Silva, J., & Coburn, J. (2021). Therapists' experience of climate change: A dialectic between personal and professional. *Counselling and Psychotherapy Research*, *23*, 417–431. Wiley (accessed on 2023).

Snyder, C. R. (2002). Hope theory: Rainbows in the mind. *Psychological Inquiry*, *13*, 249–275.

Strife, S. J. (2012). Children's environmental concerns: Expressing ecophobia. *The Journal of Environmental Education*, *43*(1), 37–54.

Thunberg, G. (2019). *Address at world economic forum*. Davos, Switzerland. 25 January 2019.

Van Susteren, L. (2021). Editorial perspective: A parable for climate collapse? *Child and Adolescent Mental Health*, *26*(3), 269–271.

Vergunst, F., & Berry, H. (2021). Climate change and children's mental health: A developmental perspective. *Clinical Psychological Science*, *10*(4), 767–785. Sage (accessed on 2022).

White, R. (2015). Imagining the unthinkable: Climate change, ecocide and children. In J. Frauley (Ed.), *C Wright Mills and the criminological imagination: Prospects for creative inquiry* (pp. 219–240). New York, NY: Routledge.

Postcards from the playroom

I once worked with a boy whose father had died very suddenly from a heart attack. Doing what she felt was best, his mother did not allow her son to see his father's body, for fear that it would be too upsetting. Soon after this, she referred him for play therapy due to his increasingly challenging behaviour, mostly anger, that was being directed towards her, for example hitting, punching and swearing.

In his sessions, I was repeatedly killed off and magically brought back to life, a pattern that continued for several weeks. Then, one day, he asked if he could use the clay. He then proceeded to make a model of what he said was his 'dead dad', lying prostrate on the ground. Temporarily banishing me to the corner of the playroom and instructing me not to look, he then sat by the clay model and said the things to his father that he not been able to say before; that he missed him and loved him. Listening to this was deeply moving. I liked him very much and he evoked a strong paternal feeling within me, perhaps an unconscious response to his intense experience of loss, connecting with aspects of my own.

In the weeks that followed, every session began with the boy asking me if I had seen his mother in the waiting area. Did I think she looked nice? Did I think she looked pretty? Did I like her? I did my best to respond congruently to these questions, but he became increasingly persistent over the following weeks, the questions growing in intensity, and I had a strong sense of where things might be leading. Until eventually;

- *Did you see my mum?*
- *Yes, I did.*
- *Did you think she looks nice? Do you like her?*
- *You are wondering if I like her. It's important to you what I think of your mum?*
- *Yes, because if you like her and think she looks nice, then you could marry her.*
- *Ah, you are wondering if I could marry your mum? Then it would be like getting your dad back again. But I am not your dad, I am your play therapist. But I understand that you really miss your dad and want him back again.*

And so there it was, the transference/countertransference breaking out into the open. We then had several sessions, together with his mother, talking about the sadness and the anger and what it is like when someone dies . . . to lose someone. In our last session, he used a polaroid camera to take pictures of us together. I still have his picture, some thirty years later, like a lost son. I didn't marry his mother, but there was a part of me that wanted to be his father.

Chapter 10

Taken

Play therapy and children in care

I have often felt something of an affinity towards children in care. I am not sure why. Being in the 'lower middle' of a family of six children, along with a large extended family from my father's previous marriage, perhaps I was never quite sure where I belonged. My parents' relationship was troubled and conflictual and I tended to absent myself, seeking solace in the natural wilderness that surrounded our rambling, country house. Perhaps it reflected something of my own internal wilderness. It was an unorthodox and unconventional childhood and as a teenager I became increasingly lost within a world that I struggled to make sense of.

Interestingly, my mother also had an affinity for children in care, and was a governor on the board of several residential schools for children with emotional and behavioural difficulties. As a teenager, I would sometimes volunteer at the EBD schools where she worked, barely older than the young people themselves. On reflection, I think there was a part of me that identified with them; that I was more like them than I cared to admit. Perhaps I was unhappier than I cared to admit. Perhaps I felt like an outsider and sought the company of other outsiders. Whatever the reasons, it was an interesting formative experience that, as discussed in Chapter 1, clearly shaped my future path.

Therapeutic work with children in care is complex and multifaceted. These are children who have in the vast majority experienced high levels of deprivation and developmental, relational trauma and who, by definition, often have had troubled, anxious and disorganised attachment histories. My experience is that these are children and young people with difficulties around emotional regulation and physical/emotional proximity, in the sense that they want to be close but are afraid to be near – the 'frightened frightening' one might say. It is a relational, attachment paradox that can see children utilising a range of defensive strategies, for example aggression, rejection, withdrawal or compliance, to keep people at a distance whilst a part of them at the same time seeks closeness and intimacy. As such, these are children with multiple deprivations; the loss of birth families and siblings and often several subsequent family placements, alongside the ongoing losses around emotional connection. Children also enter care, be it residential, foster care or adoption, due to a range of diverse reasons, often as a result of trauma and abuse but also sometimes as a result of illness, death, abandonment or complex family

DOI: 10.4324/9781003352563-10

reasons, but whatever the reason it can be taken as something of a given that these experiences will include elements of grief, loss and parental deprivation.

In this chapter then, I will look at some of the practice implications and challenges of working with children in care, drawing both from theory and my own clinical experience. This will include both what is happening inside the playroom and the material of the sessions, but also the external, systemic complexities that can impact upon the work. People will often talk of the care 'system'. It is a peculiar term that in one sense depersonalises and distances the individual experience of children who enter care, but in another sense does something to capture the complex organisational networks that surround these children. But again it is something of a proximal paradox, oscillating between the personal and professional and mirroring aspects of the child's experience. I will aim within this chapter to look at some of these organisational dynamics and how they might impact upon our work as therapists.

Some thoughts on language

During my career as a social worker, dramatherapist and play therapist, I have worked primarily within the statutory, social care sector, navigating the fine line between family support and family protection. Consequently, much of my work as a therapist has been with children and young people who have been through the care 'system', for want of a better word, as explained earlier. This includes children in both short- and long-term alternative care, foster families or children's homes, and children who have been adopted. Of course, not all children go through care; some stay in it. During the course of this work, I have often been struck by the language of children's care. We might talk about placements, transitions, respite, breakdowns and children being removed or accommodated. It is the professional vernacular; words used to sanitise and distance. In contrast, I have worked with young people who have spoken in the much more visceral terms of being 'taken', 'stolen', 'ripped' or 'torn' from their birth families. Conversely, adopted children will talk of being claimed, chosen or found. The term 'looked after' feels something of a misnomer, with children often being retraumatised by the care system itself, whilst for other children it represents a place of safety and security.

The language of care is complicated, often politicised and professionalised, a language sometimes at odds with the reality of young people's lived experience. But as is ever the case, language changes and evolves, as in the debate between *positive* and *honest* adoption language and the discussions around terms like *birth parent*, *natural parent* or *first parent*. But within this context of changing language, the guiding principle must be to ask the young people themselves; what are the words that they use, that make sense to them and reflect the reality of their own experience?

Language is important; it matters. As Blakemoore et al suggest, 'language can be one of the central factors in institutionalising environments' (2023: 18). The words we use both shape and reflect our beliefs, values and attitudes, and ultimately inform our practice. Returning to the themes of power and privilege discussed elsewhere in this book, it is important to acknowledge that children in care are a socially, emotionally (and economically) marginalised and disadvantaged 'group', experiencing high levels of stigma and shame. In this context, it is important that the language we use, our conceptual lens, does not reinforce and compound these feelings of marginalisation. Words influence how we characterise children (and subsequently how they feel characterised by others) and even the process of how to title this chapter became something of a challenge. That said, I will throughout this chapter use the term *children in care*, because it is both a term in common usage and one that broadly includes all aspects of children's care experiences, from children in foster care, children in residential group care and, to an extent, children who have been adopted, acknowledging, of course, that whilst adopted children are living in long-term, post-care families, most have had early experiences of being in care.

But it is all too easy to slip into the jargonistic language of the 'looked after' system, and we need to be mindful that this language does not oppress or discriminate. Fricker (2007) spoke of the term 'epistemic injustice', highlighting the discrimination and discreditation of those individuals, who through internalised self-labelling are unable to articulate and make sense of their experiences, or more to the point are unjustly given less credence as tellers of their own stories. This can be a particular issue for children in care in the sense that the terminology used to characterise or identify these children can reinforce the negative and harmful preconceptions that they are subjected to. As Fieller and Loughlin (2022) say,

> looked after children have been omitted from the general equality debate by both individuals and institutions. This discrimination is so deeply imbedded within the care system that the Local Authority is the only parent in England that never faces the threat of legal action for failing to protect children.
>
> (2022: 872)

For therapists, the issue of language is also important. A consequence of children in care feeling marginalised is that they can also lose their voice within the dense complexities of the child care system. This does not just create barriers to communication, but also barriers to disclosure; important for children who by the very definition of being in care have experienced acute levels of neglect and abuse. Intrinsic to this is the notion of trust, and so therapists working with children in care are in a very rarefied and privileged role of empowering them to be able to express, explore and articulate their experiences, essentially to feel heard. Therapists then, as influential advocates, can play a valuable role in countering this epistemic injustice and giving meaningful credence to children's life stories.

The baby who was never satisfied

Sophie was a 7-year-old girl, adopted at the age of 5 after spending time in two previous foster families. She had experienced chronic neglect and abuse within her birth family, and was placed in care following an emergency police protection order. She was certainly one of the most overtly traumatised children I have worked with, prone to extreme episodes of dissociation to the extent that on being placed in care she had been misdiagnosed with epilepsy. Latterly she was reassessed and her presentation recognised within the dissociative context of developmental trauma.

In the playroom, Sophie is easily triggered, for example by particular sounds, smells and physical proximity. I provide a gentle running commentary as to my position and movements and it takes several weeks before I am able to sit alongside her while she plays. Due to her high levels of anxiety and the need for her to feel as safe and contained as possible, Sophie's (adoptive) mother is also present for all her sessions; sometimes as passive observer and sometimes as a more active participant. At times, Sophie becomes very dysregulated, and will run to her mother, instigating physical and emotional contact when she needs to. In this way, her mother is an important emotionally containing and regulating presence during the sessions.

Throughout her sessions, Sophie is drawn towards the small playhouse, set up in the corner of the room. She is particularly engaged with setting up the baby's bedroom, becoming preoccupied with the baby's needs; does it have enough food, milk, clothes? Is the baby safe? Again and again she asks if the baby is 'satisfied' and this becomes an important word in her stories of neglect. She plays out brief narrative sequences in which the baby is not looked after and not getting what it needs to grow and be healthy. Sometimes she feeds and feeds the baby until it is sick, and still feeds it some more. It is often at these points in her play that Sophie becomes anxious and dissociative, noticeable in her regressive behaviour, changes in voice and eye movement, self-talking and odd physical gestures and mannerisms. Sometimes she manages to self-regulate, moving back and forth between her mother and the play and sometimes playing with the sand. At other times, when I feel she is becoming too anxious and overwhelmed by her play, I intervene more directly, either by introducing another character into her story (usually a benevolent, rescuing figure), or by redirecting her play to something more grounding, for example sequential games such as Jenga or Connect 4. Sometimes her mother will read her stories or look at picture books.

I find myself deeply affected by these intense moments of play, feeling detached and disconnected, sleepy or caught up in my own internal reverie. Perhaps, as described by Valerio (2017), these are moments of 'counterdissociation'; embodied, somatic and unconscious responses to Sophie's fragmented internal world. As Valerio suggests, episodes of embodied countertransference can lead to the therapist experiencing periods of unawareness – the hope being to have 'enough active engagement with one's own unconscious process to rapidly bring this into greater awareness so that it can be worked with in the consulting room' (Valerio, 2017: 28). Between sessions, I find myself becoming very preoccupied by Sophie, a kind of emotional ingress, as aspects of her life seem to leak into mine. I worry about her. The therapeutic relationship is informed by her complex attachment patterns that seem to move between anxious, avoidant and disorganised. At times in the sessions it is as if I do not exist; I feel left and abandoned, which is interesting within the context of her early neglect. At other times our play is very relational and there is an intensity about her focus.

Often during the sessions Sophie will run to hold her mother and ask her again to tell the story of how she came into care; asking questions about what she had or did not have as a little baby and what she was like when she was first adopted. They talk very poignantly together about what a healthy baby needs – to feel 'satisfied' – and why she did not have what she needed when she was little. The narrative around coming into care is told and retold, and in this way, Sophie moves between the symbolism of her play and the reality of her experience, each informing the other. There are two picture books in the playroom about different kinds of families, and Sophie asks her mother to repeatedly read these with her. It is very moving to watch the two of them together, piecing together a coherent narrative of her journey into care and how they came to be a family together. I recall at the outset of the work feeling anxious about Sophie's capacity to engage in the sessions, due to her very high level of trauma, and also my own ability to connect with her. The way the sessions progressed was more an evolved than planned process, as the three of us found a way to be together that enabled Sophie to feel safe and contained. The presence of Sophie's mother through this work was invaluable, providing an emotionally grounding and often very literal 'touchstone' of attachment and maternal holding. Whilst her attachment was fragile, Sophie was able to use her mother as a secure base from which to play, explore and experiment, returning to safety when she needed.

Questions of timing

It is generally accepted within child-centred play therapy, and child psychotherapy in general, that children need to be living in an emotionally secure and stable environment for them to be able to positively engage in a therapeutic process. This is an important part of the referral assessment process and clearly there are important ethical considerations around the optimal time to begin therapy. Indeed, the received wisdom is that it would not be appropriate to begin therapy with a child at a point of transition or in a short-term placement, but whilst these might be important and valid contra-indicators for therapy, for children in care the situation is often less straightforward. Apart from those who have been adopted, it could be argued that children in care are always at the point of transition and it is equally important to weigh up the ethical implications of withholding therapy, for example for children in shorter-term foster placements. Hunter (1993) suggests that children in care can spend a third of their childhood waiting; for a permanent family or for therapy. This is the paradoxical state of 'permanent impermanence' that many children in care find themselves in. The care system is full of contradictions, for example those situations where a child is not moved to another placement until they have become settled enough in their current placement – finding themselves wrenched from their foster family just at the point when they are beginning to feel more secure and beginning to form positive attachments.

Therapy can help children to process the challenging transition between placements that they have to negotiate, often many times throughout their lives. By supporting both sets of carers, therapy can act as a psychological bridge between families, securing both ends whilst the child makes the crossing from one to the other, much like a precarious rope-bridge spanning the dizzying, windy heights of a rocky canyon. It is at these points of transition when children tend to be most emotionally fragile and anxious, falling back on familiar defensive behaviours and coping strategies as a way of managing their anxiety. This can include challenging patterns of behaviour, testing to the extreme the resilience of even the most experienced of carers. The child's expectation is that the bridge will break and they will fall, once again, into the raging waters below and they will (albeit unconsciously) work hard to turn this expectation into reality; the familiar being more tolerable than the unknown.

Research by Barnardo's (Smith, 2022) shows that children in care are likely to have several different social workers, often during a single year, and experience multiple moves between foster homes and children's homes. Within this context the therapist might be one of the most consistent figures in the children's lives, providing an important level of emotional continuity and consistency. That said, as Hughes (1999) suggests, we need to be mindful that psychotherapy cannot meet all the emotional needs of the child, as much as those within the professional care network might like to think it might. As Hughes states, 'children need families first and psychotherapists second' (1999: 296). In this sense, the most effective therapeutic intervention for a child in care is a stable, loving family.

So, questions of timing are complex and can be subject to many competing needs and demands, not always in the best interests of the child. The question to ask, at the initial point of referral, is why now and whose needs are being met? A child may well be in a transitionary point in their lives, most children in care always are, and as therapist we need to invoke Winnicott's spirit of 'good enough'. Conversely, therapy might not be what is required, even though it might meet the needs of the social worker, carer or teacher. I can recall many times over the years when I have experienced sometimes intense pressure to begin therapy with a child, even though my clinical assessment (and that of my supervisor) is that the timing is not in the interests of the child. This pressure of expectation can be hard to resist, but it can be helpful at these points to hold onto a sense of clinical curiosity; what is being played out within the professional network and what is this communicating about the child's experience?

Charlotte's box of horrors

Charlotte was an 8-year-old girl, subject to a care order and initially placed with a short-term foster family, whilst a longer-term placement was sought for her. She experienced significant developmental trauma and abuse throughout her early years and on being placed in foster care, presented a range of disturbed behaviour, for example hoarding food, faecal smearing, sexualised behaviour and self-harm.

She is a challenging, feisty child – old beyond her 8 years – and I like her very much although she pushes against the therapeutic limits at every opportunity, perhaps testing out at what point I might reject her, such is her experience of life. In her first session she finds a small cardboard box and pours red paint into it. She fills the box with hastily made eyeballs attached to sticks, slime, worms and all manner of scary, 'disgusting' creatures. She calls it her 'horror box' and it feels like a very powerful, embodied and symbolic representation of her internal world. Later, she forges a house out of clay; a floor, four walls and a roof but without any windows or doors. There is no way in or out.

A therapist colleague works with the foster carers to support the placement, but Charlotte's behaviour is so challenging that the placement 'breaks down' and she is moved to another family, although this lasts only for a matter of weeks and she is moved again to a residential children's home. She is also excluded from her school and is moved to another school for children with emotional and behavioural difficulties. Her social worker also leaves during this period and a new social worker is allocated. Like Charlotte's box, the professional network is creaking at the seams and threatening to fall apart. Communication is difficult, and I feel increasingly isolated as the one person who holds some degree of continuity in Charlotte's fragmented life.

In her sessions, Charlotte plays out dramatic stories about families, usually underpinned with strong themes of rejection and abandonment as she seeks to make sense of her troubled experiences. She particularly likes to regale me with (and play out) the latest adventures of Hannah Montana, from the US teen sitcom, itself a story about a teenage girl who adopts a double life as a way of maintaining her anonymity as a 'normal' teenager. It is, at heart, a story about secret identity – the external hiding the internal – and I can understand its symbolic significance for Charlotte. I am frequently called 'stupid', an 'idiot' and (most creatively) a 'dumbarse', but she is very engaged in the sessions and I am struck by her resilience and strength of character.

I work with Charlotte for many months, although her behaviour within the children's home is becoming increasingly challenging, including episodes of swallowing harmful objects, resulting in several trips to casualty. Ultimately, those at the children's home feel that they can no longer safely manage her and she is moved, at very short notice, to a specialist out of county placement. For some reason, I am not informed of her move and she arrives for her (unbeknown to me) final session extremely angry and distressed and proceeds to trash the room; breaking things, upending furniture and tipping/squeezing out sand and paint. It is a confusing time for both of us and it is only later, when I speak to the children's home, that I can make sense of her behaviour. She feels angry and betrayed, as do I, having been placed in an invidious position by the professional network. Thankfully, I manage to negotiate an extra final ending session before she moves and do my best to repair our ruptured relationship before we say goodbye. I am left with Charlotte's box of horrors and her house with no windows or doors. Sometimes there is a fine line between symbolism and reality.

Tangled webs: issues of networking

As Lanyado (2004) suggests, there can be a powerful tendency within professional networks to unconsciously enact and repeat past traumatic episodes linked to the child's experience. As with Charlotte, there can be a destructive playing out of fragmented endings as the network struggles to contain the intolerable – the box of horrors. In Charlotte's case, communication became very difficult, key decisions were not being discussed and it became hard to keep her longer-term care plan in sight. These situations are compounded by the fact that therapy with children in care takes place within the context of often very complex professional networks; child, therapist, social worker(s), carers, respite carers, birth families, independent chairs, teachers, specialist mental health professionals etc. The list goes on. The challenge for the therapist is, as Lanyado says, being able to 'face two directions at once' (2004: 97); to hold in mind both the internal process of the child's world and the complex, external systemic dynamics of the care network.

In my experience, there can often be a merging of the two, as the network finds itself entangled in the knotted threads of competing needs, wants and agendas. The care network, as with Charlotte, might act out or mirror aspects of the child's trauma, sometimes becoming fragmented and chaotic. Children in care live within very complex, relational networks and a child in foster care, like Charlotte, might well be having contact with their birth family whilst at the same time be in a process of transition to a longer-term placement or adoptive family – three families, with very different and disparate needs and each with their varying degrees of professional support. It is hard to imagine how a child is able to emotionally navigate their way through these complex, tangled webs of family and professional networks.

At the heart of these tangled networks is a child's overwhelming experience of loss, grief, rejection and often years of abuse and trauma, and just as a child might rely upon defensive strategies and coping mechanisms to avoid the pain of the intolerable, so the professional system can do the same; finding itself caught up in unconscious, collusive patterns of anxious avoidance. Risk and responsibility, like some kind of undesirable object, can be passed from one person or organisation to another, no one wanting to hold it for too long. Perhaps unsurprisingly, it is often the therapist who is left holding these feelings, becoming isolated (like the child) and within this intense emotional vacuum, therapists can feel pressured to make decisions or recommendations clearly inappropriate to their role, for example around family contact or a move of placement.

Having worked for many years as a therapist for children with problematic and harmful sexual behaviour, I was often struck by the very polarised nature of professional networks, an unconscious playing out of the victim/victimiser dichotomy. Clearly, these network dynamics will have an impact upon the therapeutic process, with the therapist having to balance a complex range of demands and pressures. If working within a team, there might be the option of a co-worker, who can support the family or carers, enabling the therapist to maintain a contained, protected therapeutic space for the child. Consultation to professionals and carers can also be invaluable, providing a reflective 'thinking space' within the care network, promoting proactive and thoughtful decision-making rather than a more reactive acting out.

At the very heart of this work is the notion of connection. In contrast with the more classical traditions of analytic psychotherapy, which viewed therapy as something that takes place in a rather more isolated, closeted space, therapy with children in care requires a much more systemic approach, often working closely alongside parents, carers, adoptive families and associated professionals. It is a process of working that needs also to model mindful, empathic connection, especially within the context of the problematic attachment histories that so define the nature of the work. For play therapists, this process of joined up, systemic practice might include other, attachment focussed interventions, for example theraplay, filial therapy or child-parent relationship therapy. Of course, this clinical systemic overview and combination of individual and family work is important and relevant within all areas of contemporary play therapy practice, but especially so, I would suggest, within the context of work with children in care.

Separation and loss

Separation and loss are defining, key characteristics of children's experience of care, both prior to care and during care. The losses are multiple; parents, siblings, houses, school, friends, pets, possessions, as well as the psychological losses around identity and a sense of belonging. There is a sense then of cumulative, compounded loss, with children often given very little opportunity to make sense of their experiences. Transitions into care are often very sudden and abrupt with children given little notice or warning of their removal. Understandably, there are often complicated safeguarding considerations around timing, depending upon the context of the child's situation, so as not to leave the child at greater risk, but it is interesting to note the study by Mitchell and Kuczynski (2010), which found that, of twenty 8–15-year-olds in foster care, the majority were told of their removal into care on the same day that it happened. This can be a pattern continued through multiple placements, with children often being given short notice of an impending move, and it often seems that professionals and carers are cautious about giving children 'too much' notice of a placement move for fear that it will distress the child and destabilise the placement. Of course, paradoxically, this only compounds the child's feelings of loss and grief and perpetuates their already fragmented patterns of attachment; making it harder for them to form secure attachments in their new family. Contrast this, for example, with the amount of preparation and support a family might give their child in anticipation of starting school.

Leitch (2022) writes of children's experience of 'ambiguous loss', defined as 'a situation of unclear loss that remains unverified and thus without resolution' (Boss, 2016: 270). This sense of ambiguous loss is seen as the most traumatic type of loss for children in care in that it generates confusing, muddled and fragmented perceptions about relationships, family, identity and belonging. As Leitch states, children are left having to 'construct their own meaning of the situation within the contradiction and confusion associated with concurrent presence and absence of a loved person' (2022: 357). The emotionally insidious nature of ambiguous loss lies in its shapeless lack of definition. It is a known unknown; children in care may or may not be having contact with their family, may not know when they will see them again or may not even know whether they are alive or dead. Unlike 'ordinary' loss, there is no certainty that a person may come back or return and be as they were once remembered and in this sense their process of grieving might become frozen, an emotional paralysis even. There is a transient sense of being both unremembered and unforgotten, which can lead to acute feelings of confusion and uncertainty as children struggle to maintain some form of narrative coherence. Understandably, this might lead to various kinds of problematic, defensive coping strategies, and there is a danger that this kind of ambiguous loss might be pathologised, for example as a conduct disorder of one kind or another.

The author and poet Lemn Sissay, in his moving book *My Name Is Why*, wrote movingly about his personal experiences of early memories and ambiguous loss. He says,

> memories in care are slippery because there's no one to recall them with as the years pass. In a few months I would be in a different home with a different set of people who had no idea of this moment.
>
> (2020)

Sissay talks about the sense of becoming invisible; the quiet depletion of self-worth and the feeling of becoming hidden in plain sight –

> family is just a set of memories disputed, resolved or recalled between one group of people over a lifetime, isn't it? And if there is no one to care enough to dispute, resolve or recall the memory, then did it happen?
>
> (2020)

Like Charlotte's house of clay, there is a sense of being frozen in time, simultaneously trapped both inside and outside of the house with no doors and windows. Memory becomes a thing of fragmentation and dissociation; as Sissay questions, 'did it happen?' Charlotte experienced multiple moves, each contributing to a continuing experience of emotional 'contradiction and confusion' and compounding her sense of disenfranchised grief; a cumulative grief that remains mostly unacknowledged, unaddressed and unprocessed. This was, I would suggest, also a dynamic played out within the professional network; an unprocessed, non-reflective and reactively driven process of decision-making, culminating in a confused and troubled ending of therapy.

The challenge for the therapist working with children in care, is to both facilitate a therapeutic space for the child in which they can begin to process their feelings of grief and loss and at the same time create a reflective, thinking and feeling space within the professional care network, making links between the child's internal world and their external reality. Therapy may not be able to resolve children's feelings of loss and grief but can help them to find ways to live alongside these feelings. Boss describes this as 'learning to hold a paradox' (2010: 141) as children begin to find ways to tell stories about their experiences of ambiguous loss; a missed parent, friend or family pet.

I recall sessions with one young child in foster care in which we talked often about his childhood family dog and how it might be feeling scared, lonely, worried, happy or excited. We could talk about the nature of his dog's emotional bonds with people, what it needed to feel safe and its sense of a 'pack' identity and confusion when things changed. The dog became synonymous with aspects of the child's experience and when we talked it seemed that we both knew what we were really talking about, even if this did not need to be consciously articulated. Therapy can support children in care through enabling them to become more tolerant and accepting that there may not always be clear answers and that the loved and longed for relationships in their lives can be both present and absent at the same time.

By working with the care network around the child, including professionals, family members and carers, therapists can help to shift the often quite fixed perception of children's problematic behaviour; to see it through a lens of ambiguous loss and grief as opposed to something more behavioural or pathological. In other words, to see the feelings beneath the behaviour and the need beneath the feeling.

Beginnings: adoption stories

Understandably, adopted children are pre-occupied (perhaps more at certain stages in their lives than others) with questions of being 'given up'. Who are my birth parents? Why did they give me away? Was I taken away? Where are they now? Do they know about me? Primal, existential questions of self and identity. Children in foster care will have questions about belonging and whether they will ever be part of a permanent, loving family. Ultimately, these are questions of origins; imagined pasts and hoped for futures. An adopted adolescent I once worked with spoke of being 'taken', conjuring up an image of being abducted or held hostage. Perhaps better to be taken than given up. His greatest fear was that he might become like his abusive birth father. My greatest sadness was that, ultimately, he did. It is something of an existential double-bind, the 'push me/pull you' conflict of simultaneously seeking distance and closeness and the struggle of identifying with a birth parent who may have been neglectful or abusive.

Like a question one does not want an answer to, the compelling desire to know about one's origins can come at some considerable cost, but for others there might be a great relief in knowing; the reality (however hard) being better than the fantasy. I have spent many sessions with young people who have been adopted, going through their files; piecing together their family history, finding answers to their questions; and if we cannot find the answer at least working out who to ask. Life maps, genograms, timelines, creative chronologies can all be a part of this process of creating a meaningful and coherent narrative and life story. Of course, not all children want to know the answers, or indeed ask the questions, but whilst an emotionally challenging process, I am often struck by children's capacity for curiosity and their desire to embrace this process. I sometimes wonder if it is us adults who are more afraid of this process than the children themselves. But returning to questions of timing, it is important that children are feeling sufficiently 'held' to be able to manage this kind of process. When appropriate, it can be important to work alongside parents either separately or jointly with their child and it is important to acknowledge that this kind of exploratory, life-story work can be as unsettling for the parents as it can be for the child.

Origin stories are also deeply rooted within popular culture, and it is fascinating to see how children are drawn to these contemporary parables of displaced children, analogous perhaps to their own experiences. I confess that as a child I was rather obsessed with the Marvel Universe and as an adult was childishly delighted when they made their conceptual leap onto the big screen. But my personal bias aside, these flawed and often not quite so super heroes are a gift to play therapy. *Spiderman*, orphaned in childhood and raised by his extended family, is plagued by guilt and insecurity. Tony Stark's *Iron Man*, adopted as a child and adapted as an adult, engineers a formidable armoured suit but is susceptible to a fragile heart condition. Wolverine, aka Logan, the traumatised, violent child of a neglectful mother and murdered father. And over in that other (lesser) world of DC Comics, there is Batman, orphaned when his parents were killed in a violent robbery and, of course, Superman, a foundling given a home by his adoptive parents. It is not surprising to see how children in therapy are drawn to these fragile, fallible heroes; archetypal portrayals of Winnicott's false self, their vulnerabilities hidden behind an often elaborately constructed defensive façade.

Beyond the realm of comics, children's literature is abundant with similar examples. The ubiquitous Harry Potter, of course, who carries the facial scar of his orphaned childhood like a brand of difference upon his forehead. Parentless, Harry is packed off to residential school, albeit of the magical variety. Lyra Belacqua, of Pullman's His Dark Materials trilogy, is abandoned by her abusive parents and raised as an adopted child by the staff of Jordans College. And going back further into the canon of children's literature, there are examples like Mary, from Hodgson Burnett's The Secret Garden, the Jungle Book's Mowgli, raised by wolves after losing his parents and, of course, the archetypal folk tales such as Cinderella and even The Ugly Duckling.

Aside from established stories, children will, of course, create their own stories through the course of their imaginative play. Interestingly, chess has become a staple of the playroom's resources during my work with adopted children. Childhood pawns are 'taken' and find themselves clustered elsewhere in little reconstituted family groups, where playful new stories begin. The usually omnipotent maternal queen is lost, only to be found again and returned to the family. Some children end up with two queens on the board; two mothers, symbolically evocative of their lived experience. Chess is a game of two families, competing for dominance, and can resonate strongly with children in care and I am struck by some of the very creative ways in which children interpret the 'rules' of the game. One child would introduce new, fantasy characters into the game, dragons and monsters, who fight for possession of the chess pieces, dragging them back to their lairs.

Whatever the story, children will find ways to explore and express their internal world. Unexpected, resurgent memories can be at times confusing and painful, and might at other times provide relief and reassurance. But origin stories will never be that far away as children endeavour to make sense of their identity. Time is like a length of elastic, stretched ever more tightly; there is always a sense of being pulled back to the beginning.

Danny was a child in long-term residential care. Since being placed in care around the age of 8 years, he had been through multiple family placements, as many as twelve, to finally become one of the 'unplaceable' children who end up spending all their teenage life in residential care. In the playroom, Danny frequently used balls of string, thread and twine to create complex, three dimensional patterns that slowly grew until they filled the room like an immense spider's web. Strangely, it was a game I used to play as a child, with my brothers, and therefore had a poignant emotional resonance. Danny would wind the string around door handles, tables, chairs, ceiling lights, anything he could find, and as the session progressed it became increasingly hard to physically negotiate this great complex weave that gradually filled the space of the playroom. As if working some fantastical, three-dimensional loom, Danny brought the phrase 'life's rich tapestry' into a vivid reality. Like laser beams, we would have to contort our way around the room, careful not to 'set them off' or create vibrations in the string that might attract some fearsome, unseen spider. In time, we would become trapped, unable to move, and when the session ended Danny would deftly pivot and limbo his way out of the room, sometimes turning off the lights on his way out, leaving me stranded, caught in the middle of his vast tangle of knotted threads.

One could not do much better than this for an image of a child's experience of a life in care.

References

Blakemoore, E., Narey, M., Tomlinson, P., & Whitwell, J. (2023). What is institutionalising for 'looked after' children and young people? *Journal of Social Work Practice, 37*(1), 17–28.

Boss, P. (2010). The trauma and complicated grief of ambiguous loss. *Pastoral Psychology, 59*(2), 137–145.

Boss, P. (2016). The context and process of theory development: The story of ambiguous loss. *Journal of Family Theory & Review, 8*(3), 269–286.

Fieller, D., & Loughlin, M. (2022). Stigma, epistemic injustice, and 'looked after children': The need for a new language. *Journal of Evaluation in Clinical Practice, 28*, 867–874.

Fricker, M. (2007). *Epistemic injustice: Power and the ethics of knowing.* Oxford: Oxford University Press.

Hughes, C. (1999). Deprivation and children in care; the contribution of child and adolescent psychotherapy. In M. Lanyado & A. Horne (Eds.), *The handbook of child and adolescent psychotherapy.* London: Routledge.

Hunter, M. (1993). The emotional needs of children in care: An overview. *Journal of Association for Child Psychology and Psychiatry, Review Section, 15*(15), 214–218.

Lanyado, M. (2004). *The presence of the therapist: Treating childhood trauma.* Hove and New York: Routledge.

Leitch, J. (2022). Learning to hold a paradox: A narrative review of how ambiguous loss and disenfranchised grief affects children in care. *Practice: Social Work in Action, 34*(5), 355–369.

Mitchell, M. B., & Kuczynski, L. (2010). Does anyone know what is going on? Examining children's lived experience of the transition into foster care. *Children and Youth Services Review, 32*(3), 437–444.

Sissay, L. (2020). *My name is why.* Edinburgh: Canongate Books.

Smith, N. (2022). *From pillar to post; how to achieve greater stability in the care system.* London: Barnardo's Publications.

Valerio, P. (2017). *Introduction to countertransference in therapeutic practice: A myriad of mirrors.* Abingdon, UK: Routledge.

Chapter 11

Autumn leaves
Reflections on endings

In the words of the novelist Kurt Vonnegut, 'so it goes' (Vonnegut, 1969: 26). I used to read a lot of Vonnegut during my teenage years. His heady, philosophical mix of political irreverence, darkly comic satire and dystopian futures appealed to my rather angst-ridden adolescent self. He often finished a paragraph with the phrase 'so it goes' – simple words that over the passing of time became something of an emotional touchstone; a personalised motto of sorts. It is a phrase that conjures up a sense of non-judgemental acceptance; that things come and go, time passes and life goes on, straddling the temporal divide of past and present with a hint of an unsaid, unknown future. Life's little three dotted ellipsis, one could say. Writing this final chapter, just a few weeks after my 60th birthday, I feel that I am indeed at something of a pause in proceedings, and although not of the grammatical variety, those three existential dots loom large, like slippery, unsteady stepping stones across unknown waters. I hesitate, weighing up the sureness of my footing before taking that next, decisive step, not knowing quite where it might lead.

In his book *Player Piano*, Vonnegut also says, 'I want to stand as close to the edge as I can without going over. Out on the edge you see all kinds of things you can't see from the centre'. A part of being a therapist also demands that act of standing on the edge, as we step into the troubled, turbulent worlds of children's trauma, fearful of being swept away – of 'going over' – and I often think that it is only through occupying this space that we get a true sense of what it feels like to be a child having to survive the minute-to-minute emotional trials of daily life. Empathy does, after all, require the capacity to experience the feelings of the child as if they were our own. Often, when talking to a parent about their child's challenging, testing behaviour, I might pause and reflect with them for a moment about how incredibly hard and exhausting it must be for their child to live each moment in that way; to have to continually defend themselves from such overwhelming anxiety. Vonnegut's words are also about perspective and that by standing on the edge you get to notice things in a different way, whilst helping others to do the same.

Writing this book has also felt like standing on the edge. It has, perhaps inevitably, been an intensely reflective and introspective process and has also, in a strange kind of way, been quite exhausting too, as I have had to step back into often quite troubled, formative periods of my early life. In Chapter 7 I explore the notion of

DOI: 10.4324/9781003352563-11

liminality, the threshold between one space and another, like standing on the precipice of something new and unknown. This is, in a sense, where I find myself now; in the autumn of both my life and career, reflecting upon what has been and what yet is to come. It is a time of transition as I begin to let go of some of those things that have been such an integral part of my professional identity; of who I was, who I am and who I will be.

To be honest, it is a period of life that I have found myself 'nudged' towards a little sooner than I would have liked, having several years ago been diagnosed with Parkinson's Disease. Even though I have written about this extensively (Le Vay, 2022) this is a sentence that it still pains me to write, the reality of the words wrestling with the denial that even now, four years on, continues to resurface. Initially, when first diagnosed, it felt like an altogether different kind of sentence, as I struggled to confront the reality of what felt like a very changed future. Once again, it is a question of perspective and as the saying goes, life turns on a sixpence, in old money. I am not sure what this would be in new money, but it is hard to put a value on the preciousness of health – until you lose it, that is. Certainly more than a sixpence.

I was diagnosed towards the end of 2019, just months before the Covid-19 pandemic and the subsequent global lockdown felt strangely serendipitous, in that it provided me with the perfect cover for my Parkinson's. I was stuck in denial, did not want to engage with the outside world and felt acutely self-conscious around the perception of my condition. It was (is) a feeling very hard to articulate, but mostly revolves around a pervasive sense of shame, in that I felt diminished, a lesser version of myself, and as is ever the case with shame all I wanted to do was hide away, which thanks to Covid I was legitimately able to do.

Emerging out of lockdown, blinking in the dazzling glare of the outside world, I was confronted by a new reality that included, amongst a range of things, the impact of my diagnosis upon my professional, therapist identity. In Chapter 6, I talk about issues of power and vulnerability within a therapeutic context and suddenly I found myself having to face a new sense of fallibility. Much as I might like to, I have never claimed to be the omnipotent therapist (who is?) and I am not sure I could trust anyone who thought they were, but I did have to think carefully about the impact of my condition on my clients and how this might be perceived, if at all. Jung (1951) speaks of the 'wounded healer' and indeed there is an intrinsic value in acknowledging one's own vulnerabilities, but I wondered what it would be like for my clients to perceive me as the 'wounded therapist'. Would I be good enough?

Of course, many therapists have had to face the challenge of illness and incapacity. It is an inevitable part of being human and even therapists, dare I say, are human. But it is perhaps this very humanity that can bring us closer to our clients, or them to us. The psychotherapist Angela Wilton movingly wrote of her own experience of illness, suggesting that the fact that she was evidently not the healthy, invulnerable, strong therapist that she was perceived to be prior to her illness, helped in fact to equalise the power balance between her and her clients, and that it was her very vulnerability that brought this about. As she states, 'my sensed powerlessness as a result of illness enabled the other in some cases to more easily have his or her power' (2001: 1). So like any challenge, there are also potential opportunities, in this case for conversations about vulnerability, fragility, fear and hope. There is at times a fine line between vulnerability and strength, perhaps different sides of the same coin – a sixpence even – and so as I have had to recalibrate my sense of therapist identity as I seek ways of being alongside my illness, there have been some interesting, inevitable shifts in the balance of the therapeutic relationship, indeed within all my relationships. So it goes.

Of stages and ages

Winnicott famously said of being a psychotherapist that 'I aim at keeping alive, keeping well, and keeping awake' (1962: 166). Hopefully, keeping alive will not be too much of a problem, but keeping both well and awake might be a little more of a challenge as those rather unwelcome intruders of age and health begin to make their presence known. Indeed, one of the advantages of private practice is being able to schedule an afternoon nap into one's daily routine. But, as I know only too well from my own diagnosis, therapists are not invulnerable to the vicissitudes of the passing years and whilst experience is an invaluable resource, woe betide the therapist who thinks there is no more to learn. As Walcott (2011) stated when reflecting upon his own process as an ageing therapist, 'knowledge is imperfect, tranquillity is sporadic, and wisdom is doubtful' (2011: 210). Those sunlit elysian uplands seem as elusive as ever, like the teasing false summits of the long-distance hiker.

In the opening chapter of this book I reflect upon therapist beginnings, those formative first steps towards becoming a therapist and the early experiences that might shape this journey. But it can be hard to untangle where one story begins and another ends, and as Ursula Le Guin (1982), another influential writer from my younger years, suggests, we inevitably find ourselves living somewhere in the middle. Whilst there is considerable literature exploring our motivations for becoming a therapist there is perhaps less so on that challenging period of letting go, where I find myself now, which is interesting given that endings, within a clinical context, are always emphasised as being such an important part of our work. Perhaps those driving forces of unmet need and troubled early attachments that shape our 'wounded healer' therapist identity make it harder to let go, for fear that we will also be letting go of a part of ourselves. I would be the first to admit to an element of narcissism within the work, albeit of the more gentle, benign variety, but in seeing something of our own image reflected in that of our clients, the ending of our clinical work may well be accompanied by complex, entangled feelings of loss, rejection and abandonment.

Maybe it is because our work as therapists is imbued with such a strong sense of our own identity that we find it hard to relinquish. Our work *is* the relationship; we are the very tools of our trade, and this can lead to a degree of emotional entanglement that can only make the process of separation, of ending, that much harder. And in this sense, there are some very particular, unique qualities about being a play therapist that can add to the challenge of letting go. I may not miss the hours of cleaning up sand, water, glue and paint or the disposing of strange, magical mixtures and potions, like some kind of hazardous waste operative. Or the endless clearing of boxes of Lego, marbles and various assorted objects that have been gleefully upended and spilled across the floor of the playroom. Or the stifling of a pained groan as my back protests against sitting on hard floors or being stretched by the demands of keeping goal in yet another critically decisive penalty shoot-out. But there is a vitality and vigour about working with young children, a sense of unfiltered, unfettered raw immediacy, which I have always found very energising. Whether playfully serious or seriously playful, I have never ceased being amazed by the capacity and breadth of the child's imagination and the wonders of the unconscious process; the creative ways that children find to explore very challenging aspects of their lives. And it would be a lie to say that this is not personally invigorating – physically, emotionally and psychologically – and that to be in touch with the inner world of the child's imagination also fulfils a need within myself, perhaps because it keeps me within reaching distance of my own childhood – something that I do not want to let go of.

And so it is with mixed feelings and something of a heavy heart that I draw this direct, clinical period of my career to a gradual close. It is a strange, transitional time of deep emotional ambivalence, which has led me to reflect at some length upon the age and stage of life that I now find myself at, as if caught somehow by surprise. As Langer (2019) states, it is a 'curious anomaly' that in a profession so dedicated to understanding people's deepest motivations, there has been scant examination as to our own motivations for continuing to practice, or indeed discontinuing. As therapists, we are raised on the belief that endings are an essential stage and indeed goal of therapy, but it seems harder to apply that principle to ourselves. Kelly and Barratt (2007) suggest that there is a strong therapeutic case for therapists to acknowledge their own ending and 'challenging the myth or wish that therapists do not retire but go on for ever' (2007: 199). If part of becoming and being a therapist is about working through our own unresolved issues, then to end means a potentially uncomfortable shifting of the therapeutic gaze. As Neil Young poignantly sings on his seminal 1972 album, *Harvest*, 'old man look at my life, I'm a lot like you were'.

A further defining aspect of being a play therapist is the age of our clients. The children remain the same age, we do not, and whilst the wonderful, magical imagination of the playroom can defy the rules of physics, of time and space, as therapists we are unfortunately unable to defy the rules of ageing. No Peter Pan or Dorian Gray; eventually the pained portrait in the attic will catch up with us as the work takes its toll. Just as we might talk about children's stages and ages, we cannot ignore our own developmental trajectory, played out as much through the unconscious process as anywhere else. The vagaries of transference and counter-transference are such that at different points along this developmental continuum,

I have as a therapist inhabited the role of sibling, parent and now, it must be said, grandparent. It is a sobering thought and, of course, children are only too quick to remind us of our impending fallibility. I have, I hope mostly with affection, been called old, boring and a dumb-arse, and much worse. I have been killed off, married off and even given birth. As I have said before, the playroom provides a magical space where anything can happen, and most things do. But as the saying goes, out of the mouth of babes, and perhaps there is a truth to be found in these playful exchanges, if one chooses to look for it.

But age also brings new and sometimes surprising qualities into the work. I have found a different kind of lightness and humour in being with children, less caught up in the angst of theory and more relaxed and considered about boundaries and limits in a way that has allowed me to be more comfortable in being myself, a kind of relaxed sense of congruence. Perhaps, like the grandparent that some children see me as, there is more generational distance, allowing space for a playful relationship free from parental worries about rules, behaviour and expectation. Maybe the children see me more as a benevolent playmate rather than figure of authority. In the real world, whilst a father I am not actually a grandparent and interestingly, I never knew any of my own grandparents, so it is a role and stage of life that feels new and unfamiliar.

The psychologist Sachs (2020) talks about his own transition into the grandfatherly years of clinical practice and how he found himself feeling more optimistic about his work and better inclined towards the families. He says, 'I am less alarmist but that I also seem able to see the strength and resilience of the human spirit being refracted more wondrously than ever before' (2020: 2017) and whilst being 'bumped up a step on humanity's generational ladder' inevitably means being confronted with one's limitations and vulnerabilities, Sachs suggests that it was this very process of having to embrace his limitations that enabled him to more effectively empathise and be present with his clients – 'precisely because they, too, are struggling with limitations and vulnerabilities' (2020: 2017).

So my retirement, if I can call it that, from clinical work has been a gradual incremental process, and feels somewhat bittersweet as I make those difficult decisions about what to hold onto and what to let go. These decisions are based upon many factors, some related to age and health but others related to a much wider context, for example issues of relationships, family and finances; these are not decisions taken in isolation. There were for me also practical considerations around clinic space and lease contracts that led me to having to make some decisions sooner than I would have liked. But as I say, whether it can be called retirement or not is a moot point, as the act of creating space in one's life also creates opportunities for other activity. I write, present, teach occasionally, supervise and keep up my twin passions of long-distance hiking and playing the piano.

That said, there are clearly losses and gains and personally it has not been an easy transitional period. For better or worse, our sense of identity and self-worth is tightly wrapped up in the familiar, patterned paper of our professional lives and when the wrapping comes loose, we might feel a little unsure as to what we will find inside; what it is that we have exactly been gifted with. Intrinsic to this is a sense of meaning; how do we as therapists replace or move on from the kind of work that has so clearly defined us? If you take away that sense of definition, what do we have left to hold us in shape? As Shatsky (2016) says, 'for many of us, the practice space is the place where we have nurtured and cultivated our most creative, risk-taking, independent selves' (2016: 149) and in this sense, it will always be a space that is hard to replace.

As a play therapist, I have felt both privileged and honoured to be able to share the rarefied, internal worlds of the children and young people that I have worked with over the years, and so in many ways the unique intimacy of the therapeutic relationship does indeed feel irreplaceable. This interdependent, mutually beneficial dynamic of therapy evokes, for want of a better expression, something of a protection racket, not in the exploitative sense but in the sense that, implicit within the contract, is the shared meeting of need. The process of ending, especially within the context of retirement, can come at some considerable emotional cost and so, as Shatsky suggests, just as the retiring therapist abandons their clients, in taking such action so we too are equally abandoned.

There are, therein, ethical issues to be considered. There are many reasons why one might decide to retire from clinical practice, matters of both choice and necessity, each with their own losses and gains, challenges and opportunities. Following my diagnosis, I had to carefully consider the ethical context of my work; issues of fitness to practice and whether I was able to continue to meet the needs of my clients. As Wilton (2001: 1) states, in order to work as a psychotherapist it is the

> responsibility of each of us to make sure we are in a fit state to do so. We must be sound enough physically and emotionally, grounded enough to be able to meet whatever our patients need to bring to us, throw at us, engage us in disentangling.

Faced with the unknown future nature of my condition and the impact it may or may not have upon my clinical practice, I had to ask myself whether I would be able to continue to fulfil the aforementioned pre-requisite. As it was, discussions both with my clinical supervisor and medical consultant were integral to this process, providing both guidance and reassurance as to how I could best manage the demands of my clinical practice.

More generally, this question of fitness to practice is one that we all need to reflect upon as we enter the autumn years of our professional lives. We will inevitably be confronted, at some time or another, with issues of illness, incapacity, infirmity, cognitive decline or simply the banal realities of ageing and we cannot assume, as is perhaps sometimes the case within the therapy profession, that we are immune to the effects of the advancing years and can work to an open-ended, limitless timescale. We cannot, or should not, go on forever. Equally, we might want to avail ourselves of the opportunities that life brings beyond our professional lives; travel, creative expression, family relationships and the exploration of new skills. But as Shatsky reminds us, 'everything, including the therapeutic relationship, ends. This can never be well timed. However, preparation for that inevitability is an imperative responsibility of ethical practice' (2016: 149).

Of politics and polemics

Beyond matters of health and age, one of the other things that I have been struck by through writing this book is the recurrent, interconnected themes that run through the chapters. Perhaps I should not be surprised by this. Questions of childhood, self-doubt, power, vulnerability, politics and social justice have been ever-present, I guess because they have all been an important part of my personal and professional identity. I am also aware that I have transgressed the convention of therapist neutrality and been relatively forthcoming in terms of my views and opinions. In fact, I am unsure there is such a thing as therapist neutrality, the question being how we balance our personal values and attitudes with the core non-judgemental conditions of child-centred play therapy.

And as I think has been all too clear, I do not find it easy to separate the personal from the political from the professional, and indeed I wonder to what extent I should. It sounds like a cliché, but we live in challenging, unprecedented times, as matters of war, climate change, pollution and social injustice press upon us more than ever. Intersectional, societal fault lines have not just been laid bare, but riven and torn asunder by the resurgent forces of populism that ever polarise an already fractured society. Just today, as I write this, we are told that the UK has lost almost half of its natural biodiversity, whilst at the same time the government announces the opening-up of vast, new oilfields off the coast of Scotland and the number of unaccompanied children making perilous boat journeys across the Mediterranean has risen by 60%. These things are not unrelated, and my personal responses to these uncomfortable facts are a result of political held values and attitudes that not everyone will choose to share, which is fine, but which are a part of who I am; an expression of my personal, social and political identity.

The question is how, as therapists, we should respond to such challenges, if at all. Do we have a social, ethical, moral responsibility to address, acknowledge, question or even challenge matters of social justice within the context of our work? As citizens of an interconnected world, I would suggest that there is a collective responsibility to address these issues, to contribute what we can both in terms of our individual practice but also more systemically across our respective professional and governing bodies. If anything, therapy is about connection and where there is connection there is hope, and where there is hope there is agency. We cannot ignore the fact that we are working within a political context that impacts upon the day to day lives of our clients, but that said, being a politically informed therapist does not mean the imposition of our belief system or the adopting of a particular political position, whatever that may be. But it might mean being more open and congruent about one's own values, attitudes, beliefs and morals; to be responsive to the worries and anxieties that children and their families are experiencing and to facilitate a safe space within which these feelings can be explored.

Inevitably, children bring their anxieties into their sessions, the reality of the external world crashing in on the protected, symbolic space of the playroom and breaching the defences of the therapeutic boundary. As seen by myself and many of my colleagues, the emergent themes of the climate crisis and international conflict have begun to become more visible within children's play, whilst externally the pressures of austerity and the cost-of-living crisis impacts the lives of the families we are working with. Whatever the nature of our political beliefs, these are the realities within which we are working. Perhaps we can understand Winnicott's desire to stay *alive*, *well* and *awake* beyond its literal meaning; in that we need to remain alert, receptive and attuned to our client's needs, dilemmas and concerns within the context of the socio-political world in which we live.

Kicking up the leaves

It's October, perhaps my favourite month, and like most days I go for a walk for a few miles around the local woods and common land close to where I live. The woods are mixed in nature, part open heathland and part woodland, mainly coniferous but also liberally laced with beech, oak, chestnut and silver birch, amongst others. The mixture of peaty, acidic soil and the damp, heavy soil of the local clay beds provide a rich, earthy foundation for grassland, scrub, areas of marsh and in places dense woodland. Today is a nice morning and I feel gently heated by the welcome, rising warmth of the autumn sun. The night's rain hangs heavy in the air and engenders a reflective stillness to the scene, a little mournful perhaps, whilst the beautifully pungent, pervasive, moss-infused ether permeates my senses. With the woodland canopy lit by the thin morning sunlight, the autumnal, impressionistic spectrum from pale yellow-green to the darkest of brown is spectacular; a chromatic, spectral wonderland so intense that it evokes, if such thing is possible, a subdued sense of psychedelia, so vivid and powerful are the trees colouring.

The ground is thickly layered with fallen leaves and every now and again I walk through the half-plundered and scattered remains of chestnut shells that lie camouflaged like spiky sea urchins upon an ocean bed. The grass, bramble and bracken-bedecked borders of the path are delicately embroidered with silvery spiders' webs, and being as yet untouched by the early sun are still coated with the morning's crystalline dew. Curious, I search briefly for the elusive spiders responsible for these fragile constructions but they remain safely hidden away as they await the tell-tale tug of a careless insect that has become ensnared in their sticky strands of silk. Every now and again along the path, toadstools push up through the wet leaves, lending their own transient magic to the scene. Some of them stand proud with their large, white parasols open for inspection whilst others, small and brown, sit gently unseen amongst the turning leaves. Following the gently flowing, meandering course of the river Mole that has been such a steadfast companion over the years, I am (if lucky) rewarded by the startling, electric blue flash of a kingfisher. One of nature's many gifts.

Autumn is a reflective time of the year, as the days shorten and the light thins, and it is by timely happenstance that I find myself writing the final chapter of this book in mid-October. When I walk, beguiled by the gently dissociative, immersive quality of the natural world, I often find myself reflecting upon the period of my life that I now find myself in. My career, like so many paths, has been a rather circuitous journey, not so much a conscious plan but more the winding ramble of one of my many woodland walks; not knowing quite where I am going or how I am going to get there. Sometimes we are surprised by our eventual destination; in the words of David Byrne and the seminal band Talking Heads, 'you may ask yourself, well how did I get here?' It is something I have asked myself many times. As I look back now and reflect upon the route that has led me here, I can see that it has made a kind of sense and as I have spoken about in Chapter 2, the pieces of the jigsaw puzzle, the training, theory and practice, have somehow come together to form a near complete picture, even if it was not the one on the front of the box, assuming there ever was a box in the first place. Like a jigsaw, I was never sure if I was working in from the outside or out from the inside. To paraphrase a certain Eric Morecombe, *all the right pieces, but not necessarily in the right order*. Perhaps this is the process that lies at the heart of integrative practice, in that we eventually find a way to fit the pieces together to form a coherent understanding that feels unique and meaningful to each of us. There is no right order; we have to discover an order that feels right for us.

I began this book by talking about our pathways into training and beyond; those early childhood influences and drives that might motivate us to train as therapists. Now I find myself reflecting upon the autumn, twilight years of my therapeutic career. Recently, I made the decision, along with colleagues, to close our jointly run practice that has been our clinic space for many years. It was a strange experience; clearing the room, removing the furniture and taking down pictures. I spent hours sifting and sorting; going through boxes of objects, sandplay miniatures, stones, shells and figures. I emptied out my sandtray, cleared out pots of pens, paint, glue, books and games. And of course, like Aladdin's Lamp, everything I dusted, cleaned or threw away conjured up genies from the past, a spectral evocation of the many children that I have worked with in this room over the years. Every object was infused with the remembered spirit of one child or another; a story, a sequence of play, a game played. Kicking through the fallen leaves of my career, I was surprised by the feelings uncovered; the joy, pleasure, sadness, relief. And throughout this was a deep sense of ambivalence as I questioned whether I was doing the right thing. There was a feeling of something unfinished, as I sifted through the fragments of the puzzle, looking for that ever-elusive missing piece.

Our work defines us, for better and worse, and being a therapist, trainer and lecturer has for so long held my sense of personal identity, a course shaped and patterned by the narrative flow of the passing years, much like the eroded, meandering course of my old friend the river Mole. As I gradually step away from the familiar comfort of my professional self, I am confronted with that uncomfortable thought of what I used to be, the missing piece. What do I tell people now when they ask me what I do for a living? Boyd-Carpenter, reflecting upon her own retirement from clinical practice, said that, 'part of engaging in any activity or any relationship is to have knowledge from the outset of its end and of the layers of loss that will one day come' (2010: 89). Yes, there are losses, that will one day come, but there are also gains. Those years of experience are not lost, rather they become an integral part of what we are now, and what we will become. Leaves might fall, but only to allow new ones to grow. Perhaps there is no missing piece; this is who I am.

A new day, and as I look out of the window the rain clears and the sun gently pushes its way through the grey, October clouds. Time to go for a walk.

References

Boyd-Carpenter, M. J. (2010). Reflections on retirement. *Psychodynamic Practice, 16*(1), 89–94.

Jung, C. (1951). *Fundamental questions of psychotherapy*. Princeton, NJ: Princeton University Press.

Kelly, M., & Barratt, G. (2007). Retirement: Phantasy and reality: Dying in the saddle or facing up to it? *Psychodynamic Practice, 13*(2), 197–202.

Langer, R. (2019). Psychotherapist retirement: What is lost and what is gained. *Psychodynamic Practice, 25*(4), 342–355. https://doi.org/10.1080/14753634.2019.1670094.

Le Guin, U. (1982). *The left hand of darkness*. London: Orbit.

Le Vay, D. (2022). *Personal process in child-centred play therapy*. London: Routledge.

Sachs, B. (2020). *The good enough therapist*. New York: Routledge.

Shatsky, P. (2016). Everything ends: Identity and the therapist's retirement. *Clinical Social Work Journal, 44*, 143–149.

Vonnegut, K. (1969). *Slaughterhouse-five*. New York: Delacorte Press.

Walcott, W. (2011). Reflections on retirement. *Psychological Perspectives, 54*(2), 208–225. https://doi.org/10.1080/00332925.2011.573388.

Wilton, A. (2001). The impact of illness on the therapist's self and the handling and use of this in therapy. *Reformulation, ACAT News Autumn*, x.

Winnicott, D. (1962). The aims of psycho-analytical treatment. In *The maturational processes and the facilitating environment*. London: Hogarth. (Original work published 1965).

Index

For Product Safety Concerns and Information please contact our EU
representative GPSR@taylorandfrancis.com Taylor & Francis Verlag GmbH,
Kaufingerstraße 24, 80331 München, Germany

Printed and bound by CPI Group (UK) Ltd, Croydon, CR0 4YY
08/06/2025
01897005-0017